ASH-SAP American Society of Hematology Self-Assessment Program

SECOND EDITION

Editors

Michael E. Williams, MD
Marc J. Kahn, MD

Chapter Authors

Thomas Abshire, MD
Virginia C. Broudy, MD
George R. Buchanan, MD
Michael A. Caligiuri, MD
Bruce M. Camitta, MD
Spero R. Cataland, MD
Mark Crowther, MD, MSC, FRCPC
Barbara Degar, MD
John J. Densmore, MD, PhD
James N. George, MD
Jay H. Herman, MD
Meghan A. Higman, MD, PhD
Ronald Hoffman, MD
Carol Ann Huff, MD
Marc J. Kahn, MD
Thomas R. Klumpp, MD
Cindy Leissinger, MD
Michael Linenberger, MD
Richard Lottenberg, MD
Chadi Nabhan, MD
Pierre Noel, MD
Robert E. Richard, MD, PhD
Margaret E. Rick, MD
Daniel Rosenblum, MD, FACP
Yogen Saunthararajah, MD
Kevin Shannon, MD
Kimberly Stegmaier, MD
F. Marc Stewart, MD
Martin S. Tallman, MD
Georgia B. Vogelsang, MD
Michael E. Williams, MD
Ted Wun, MD, FACP
Marc Zumberg, MD

Published by

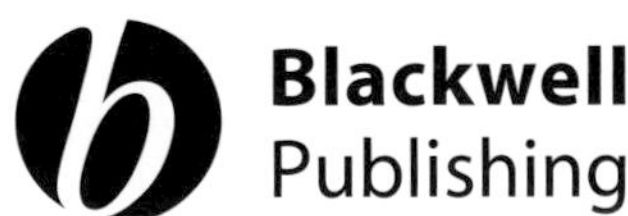

American Society of Hematology
1900 M Street N.W., Suite 200
Washington, DC 20036
202-776-0544

First published 2003 by Blackwell Publishing
Second edition 2005
Blackwell Publishing, Inc., 350 Main Street, Malden, Massachusetts 02148-5020, USA
Blackwell Publishing Ltd, 9600 Garsington Road, Oxford OX4 2DQ, UK
Blackwell Publishing Asia Pty Ltd, 550 Swanston Street, Carlton, Victoria 3053, Australia

ISBN 1-4051-2705-8

Catalogue records for this title are available from the Library of Congress and the British Library

Set in 10/13pt Minion by Graphicraft Limited, Hong Kong
Printed and bound by Walsworth Publishing Company, Marceline, Missouri, USA

For further information on Blackwell Publishing, visit our website:
http://www.blackwellpublishing.com

Contents

© Dennis Kunkel Microscopy, Inc

Authors

© Dennis Kunkel Microscopy, Inc

Thomas Abshire, MD
Professor of Pediatrics
Director, Comprehensive Hemophilia Program
AFLAC Cancer Center and Blood Disorders Service
Emory University
Atlanta, Georgia

Virginia C. Broudy, MD
Chief of Medicine
Harborview Medical Center
Professor and Vice Chair
Department of Medicine
University of Washington
Seattle, Washington

George R. Buchanan, MD
Professor of Pediatrics
Children's Cancer Fund Distinguished Chair in Pediatric Oncology and Hematology
University of Texas Southwestern Medical Center at Dallas
Dallas, Texas

Michael A. Caligiuri, MD
Director, Comprehensive Cancer Center
Deputy Director, Arthur G. James Cancer Hospital and Richard J. Solove Research Institute
Director, Division of Hematology and Oncology
Department of Internal Medicine,
College of Medicine and Public Health
Columbus, Ohio

Bruce M. Camitta, MD
Director, Midwest Children's Cancer Center
Rebecca Jean Slye Professor of Pediatric Oncology
Medical College of Wisconsin
Children's Hospital of Wisconsin
Milwaukee, Wisconsin

Spero R. Cataland, MD
Clinical Assistant Professor of Internal Medicine
Division of Hematology and Oncology
Ohio State University
Columbus, Ohio

Mark Crowther, MD, MSc, FRCPC
Associate Professor of Medicine
Director, Hematology Residency Training Program
McMaster University
Head of Service, Hematology
St Joseph's Hospital
Hamilton, Ontario, Canada

Barbara Degar, MD
Attending Physician, Dana Farber Cancer Institute and Children's Hospital Boston
Instructor in Pediatrics, Harvard Medical School
Boston, Massachusetts

John J. Densmore, MD, PhD
Assistant Professor of Clinical Internal Medicine
University of Virginia School of Medicine
Charlottesville, Virginia

James N. George, MD
Professor of Medicine
Hematology-Oncology Section
University of Oklahoma Health Sciences Center
Oklahoma City, Oklahoma

Jay H. Herman, MD
Clinical Professor
Departments of Medicine and Anatomy, Pathology and Laboratory Medicine
Director of Transfusion Medicine
Associate Director for Education
Cardeza Foundation for Hematologic Research
Thomas Jefferson University
Philadelphia, Pennsylvania

Meghan A. Higman, MD, PhD
Assistant Professor of Oncology and Pediatrics
The Sidney Kimmel Comprehensive Cancer Center at Johns Hopkins
Baltimore, Maryland

Ronald Hoffman, MD
Professor of Medicine and Chief, Section of Hematology/Oncology
Department of Medicine
University of Illinois-Chicago
Chicago, Illinois

Carol Ann Huff, MD
Assistant Professor
Department of Oncology
Sidney Kimmel Comprehensive Cancer Center at Johns Hopkins University
Baltimore, Maryland

Marc J. Kahn, MD
Professor of Medicine
Associate Dean for Student Affairs
Tulane University School of Medicine
New Orleans, Louisiana

Thomas R. Klumpp, MD
Associate Professor of Medicine
Temple University School of Medicine
Assistant Director
Fox Chase-Temple University Bone Marrow Transplant Program
Philadelphia, Pennsylvania

Cindy Leissinger, MD
Professor of Medicine, Pediatrics and Pathology
Director, Louisiana Center for Bleeding and Clotting Disorders

Tulane University Health Sciences Center
New Orleans, Louisiana

Michael Linenberger, MD
Medical Director, Apheresis and Cellular Therapy, Seattle Cancer Care Alliance
Associate Professor of Medicine, University of Washington
Associate Member, Fred Hutchinson Cancer Research Center
Seattle, Washington

Richard Lottenberg, MD
Professor of Medicine
Division of Hematology/Oncology
Department of Medicine
University of Florida School of Medicine
Gainesville, Florida

Chadi Nabhan, MD
Oncology Specialists, S.C.
Lutheran General Hospital Cancer Center
Clinical Assistant Professor
Northwestern University Feinberg School of Medicine
Park Ridge, Illinois

Pierre Noel, MD
Chief Hematology Section, Division of Laboratory Medicine
NIH Clinical Center
Bethesda, Maryland

Robert E. Richard, MD, PhD
Assistant Professor
Division of Hematology, Department of Medicine
University of Washington School of Medicine
Seattle, Washington

Margaret E. Rick, MD
Assistant Chief, Hematology Service
Warren Grant Magnuson Clinical Center
National Institutes of Health
Bethesda, Maryland

Daniel Rosenblum, MD, FACP
Division of Clinical Evaluation and Pharmacology/Toxicology
Office of Cellular, Tissue and Gene Therapies
Center for Biologics Evaluation and Research
US Food and Drug Administration
Rockville, Maryland

Yogen Saunthararajah, MD
Assistant Professor
Section of Hematology/Oncology
University of Illinois at Chicago
Chicago, Illinois

Kevin Shannon, MD
Professor of Pediatrics
University of California
Hematopoietic Malignancies Program Leader
UCSF Comprehensive Cancer Center
San Francisco, California

Kimberly Stegmaier, MD
Attending Physician, Dana Farber Cancer Institute and Children's Hospital Boston
Instructor in Pediatrics, Harvard Medical School
Boston, Massachusetts

F. Marc Stewart, MD
Medical Director, Seattle Cancer Care Alliance
Professor of Medicine, University of Washington
Member, Fred Hutchinson Cancer Research Center
Seattle, Washington

Martin S. Tallman, MD
Professor of Medicine
Division of Hematology-Oncology
Department of Medicine
Northwestern University Feinberg School of Medicine
Co-Director, Hematologic Malignancy Program
Robert H. Lurie Comprehensive Cancer Center
Chicago, Illinois

Georgia B. Vogelsang, MD
Professor of Oncology
Johns Hopkins University School of Medicine
Baltimore, Maryland

Michael E. Williams, MD
Byrd S. Leavell Professor of Medicine and Professor of Pathology
Director, Hematologic Malignancy Program
Hematology/Oncology Division and Cancer Center
University of Virginia School of Medicine
Charlottesville, Virginia

Ted Wun, MD, FACP
Associate Professor of Medicine
Associate Chief and Fellowship Program Director
Division of Hematology/Oncology, UC Davis SOM
Chief, Section of Hematology and Oncology
VA Northern California Health Care System
Sacramento, California

Marc Zumberg, MD
Assistant Professor
Medical Director, Therapeutic Apheresis, LifeSouth
Department of Medicine, University of Florida
Division of Hematology/Oncology
Gainesville, Florida

CME information

Accreditation

The American Society of Hematology designates this educational activity for a maximum of 50 category 1 credits toward the AMA Physician's Recognition Award.

The American Society of Hematology designates this educational activity for a maximum of **50** hours of category 1 credit toward the AMA Physician's Recognition Award. Each physician should claim only those hours of credit that he/she actually spent in the educational activity.

Target audience

ASH-SAP is a high-quality educational product offering up-to-date information in the field of hematology for hematologists, medical oncologists, internists, pediatricians and hematology-oncology fellows and trainees.

Educational objectives

This program includes a printed syllabus divided into chapters dedicated to specific topical areas in hematology, as well as a self-assessment test composed of case-based, multiple-choice questions and critiques. A web-based multimedia component reflecting the same information contained in the printed text, but adding an interactive element to the self-assessment, is also included.

The self-assessment's goals are:

1 to provide timely clinical updates on new developments in hematology

2 to help practicing physicians prepare for recertification

3 to serve as a tool for board review

Date of release:
December 1, 2004

Disclosure

As a provider accredited by the Accreditation Council for Continuing Medical Education (ACCME), the American Society of Hematology must insure balance, independence, objectivity, and scientific rigor in all of its individually-sponsored and jointly-sponsored educational activities. All faculty participating in a sponsored activity are expected to disclose to the activity audience any significant financial interest or other relationship (1) with the manufacturer(s) of any commercial product(s) and/or provider(s) of commercial services discussed in an educational presentation and (2) with any commercial supporters of the activity. *(Significant financial interest or other relationship can include such things as grants or research support, employee, consultant, major stock holder, member of speakers bureau, etc.)* The intent of this disclosure is not to prevent a speaker with a significant financial or other relationship from making a presentation, but rather to provide listeners with information on which they can make their own judgments. It remains for the audience to determine whether the speaker's interests or relationships may influence the presentation with regard to exposition or conclusion.

	Research support/ Research	Consultant	Major stockholder	Speakers' bureau	Scientific Advisory Board
Thomas Abshire		Novo Nordisk, Bayer, Baxter, Wyeth, ZLB Behring		Novo Nordisk, Bayer, Baxter, Wyeth, ZLB Behring	
Virginia C. Broudy	Amgen	Amgen			
George R. Buchanan					
Michael A. Caligiuri					
Bruce M. Camitta				Sanofi-Synthelabo Inc.	
Spero R. Cataland					
Mark Crowther	Leo Laboratories, Aventis/Sanofi, Pfizer/Pharmacia	Bayer, Leo Laboratories, Aventis/Sanofi, Pfizer/ Pharmacia, Astra Zeneca		Leo Laboratories, Aventis/Sanofi, Pfizer/ Pharmacia, Calea	
Barbara Degar					
John J. Densmore	BiogenIDEC, Celgene			BiogenIDEC, Genentech	
James N. George		Amgen			
Jay H. Herman				Health Learning Systems (Berlex)	
Meghan A. Higman					
Ronald Hoffman					
Carol Ann Huff					
Marc J. Kahn					
Thomas R. Klumpp					
Cindy Leissinger					
Michael Linenberger					
Richard Lottenberg					
Chadi Nabhan					
Pierre Noel					
Robert E. Richard					
Margaret E. Rick					
Daniel Rosenblum					
Yogen Saunthararajah					
Kevin Shannon	Merck Pfizer	Onyx, Plexikom			Nexgenix
Kimberly Stegmaier					
F. Marc Stewart					
Martin S. Tallman	Cell Therapeutics Inc., Wyeth Oncology	Cell Therapeutics Inc., Wyeth Oncology		Cell Therapeutics Inc., Wyeth Oncology	Cell Therapeutics Inc., Wyeth Oncology
Georgia B. Vogelsang					
Michael E. Williams	BiogenIDEC, Salmedix, Genentech	Genentech, BiogenIDEC		Genentech, BiogenIDEC, Berlex	
Ted Wun					
Marc Zumberg					

In compliance with ACCME policy, the American Society of Hematology requires its faculty to disclose to the activity audience any discussion of off-label use of a drug or medical device in their presentations.

The following authors disclosed these off-label uses in their materials:

Dr. Broudy's chapter will discuss other, non-FDA-approved uses of growth factors. In each case, the non-FDA-approved uses are labeled "other uses" or "potential uses."

Dr. Klumpp will discuss Amicar for prophylaxis of bleeding in thrombocytopenic patients.

Dr Linenberger will discuss the off-label use of therapeutic agents used for rare disorders.

Dr. Lottenberg will discuss Rituximab and IVIG for autoimmune hemolytic anemia.

In Dr. Vogelsang's chapter, all mentions of drugs will be off-label.

Dr. Williams will discuss front-line Rituximab, combined chemotherapy and Rituximab, Rituximab in CLL.

Dr. Densmore will discuss thalidomide and derivatives in myeloma.

Dr. Wun will discuss some off-label use of low molecular weight heparins.

Getting credit

In order to receive AMA category 1 credit for participation in this educational activity, you must first complete the self-assessment test located in the accompanying test booklet, or you may complete the test online on the companion website. Scores of 80% or better are eligible to claim credit for the activity.

If you complete the test in the booklet, mail your completed test sheet to:

American Society of Hematology
Continuing Medical Education Department
1900 M Street N.W., Suite 200
Washington, DC 20036

Instructions for obtaining credit after completing the test online are found on the companion website. Participants may claim CME credit for completing this edition of the SAP program until December 2007.

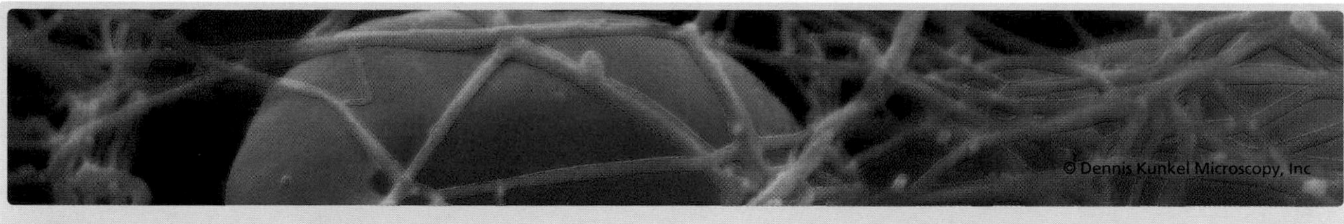

Questions

Question 1

A 16-year-old female presents with bruising and petechiae after a several month history of lower back pain. She has marked splenomegaly on physical examination. Complete blood count shows WBC of 80 K with circulating blasts, anemia and thrombocytopenia. Flow cytometry shows a population of cells that are terminal deoxynucleotidyl transferase-positive (TdT^+), $CD10^+$, $CD19^+$, T-cell and myeloid marker negative. Cytogenetics demonstrates the presence of the t(9;22).

Q Which of the following studies would support the diagnosis of chronic myeloid leukemia with lymphoid blast crisis in this patient?

A Genomic polymerase chain reaction (PCR) demonstrating the presence of p210
B Western blot demonstrating the presence of p190
C Fluorescence *in situ* hybridization (FISH) studies confirming the presence of the t(9;22)
D Reverse transcriptase PCR (RT-PCR) studies demonstrating the presence of the p210 transcript

Question 2

A 55-year-old male presents with shortness of breath on exertion and fatigue. His complete blood count (CBC) results include: hemoglobin 7 g/dL, absolute reticulocyte count 50×10^9/L, white blood cell count 1.0×10^9/L, absolute neutrophil count 0.5×10^9/L and platelets 23×10^9/L. The mean corpuscular volume is 96 fL. Bone marrow trephine biopsy is hypocellular with abnormal localization of immature precursors (ALIPs).

Q The most likely diagnosis is:

A Severe aplastic anemia
B Folate deficiency
C Hypoplastic myelodysplastic syndrome
D B_{12} deficiency

Question 3

A 41-year-old man is found to be HIV-positive with a CD4 count of 112/μL and a viral load of 300,000 copies/mL. He complains of easy bruising. He has not had nose bleeding or gum bleeding. His complete blood cell count (CBC) is white blood cell count (WBC) 4500/μL, HCT 34%, platelets 15,000/μL. His peripheral smear shows normal WBC and red blood cell (RBC) morphology, and confirms a decreased number of platelets.

Q (a) What is the most likely cause of this patient's thrombocytopenia?

A Vitamin B_{12} deficiency
B Thrombotic thrombocytopenic purpura (TTP)
C Marrow failure resulting from HIV
D Idiopathic thrombocytopenic purpura (ITP)

Q (b) Which of the following is the most appropriate management for this patient?

A Start oprelvekin (IL-11)
B Start highly active antiretroviral therapy
C Prompt splenectomy
D Platelet transfusion
E Start vitamin B_{12} therapy

Question 4

A 39-year-old woman presents with extreme fatigue and decreased exercise tolerance. She has no significant medical history and has been taking natural products, including ginseng, garlic and turmeric as health supplementation. Two years ago she had an upper respiratory infection and also began taking ascorbic acid, echinacea and zinc lozenges. Even though her viral symptoms resolved, she continued to take these medications indefinitely. She now begins to experience extreme fatigue and decreased exercise tolerance. The physical examination is significant for pallor and tachycardia. She is found to have a hemoglobin of 8.0 g/dL with a mean corpuscular volume (MCV) of 67 fL.

Q Which of the following medications is the most likely cause for her anemia?

A Ginseng
B Turmeric
C Ascorbic acid
D Echinacea
E Zinc

Question 5

A 7-year-old girl is found to be anemic with a hemoglobin of 9 mg/dL and a mean cell volume (MCV) of 68 fL. She is also noted to have a ferritin of 9 μg/dL and serum iron of 25 μg/dL. Her parents report her to have a normal diet. She is evaluated for blood loss with endoscopy and is found to have a grossly normal esophagus, stomach, duodenum and colon. Gastric biopsies are positive for *Helicobacter pylori* without inflammation. Oral ferrous sulfate replacement is begun, which does not result in reticulocytosis or resolution of her anemia.

Q Which of the following interventions is most appropriate to resolve her anemia?

A Eradicate *H. pylori* infection
B Begin parenteral cobalamin therapy
C Begin folate therapy
D Change her iron supplementation to ferrous fumarate
E Change her iron supplementation to ferrous gluconate

Question 6

A 45-year-old male with severe alcoholic liver disease is referred to you for pretransplant evaluation of anemia that has become more severe over the past 3 months. During this period he has been treated for encephalopathy and refractory ascites. He is known to have esophageal varices, but has had no evidence of gastrointestinal bleeding. Results of laboratory data and peripheral smear (see Figure) are shown below:

Hematocrit	24%
WBC count	3700/μL
Platelet count	107,000/μL
Reticulocyte count	9%
Bilirubin, total	6.5 mg/dL
Bilirubin, direct	1.9 mg/dL

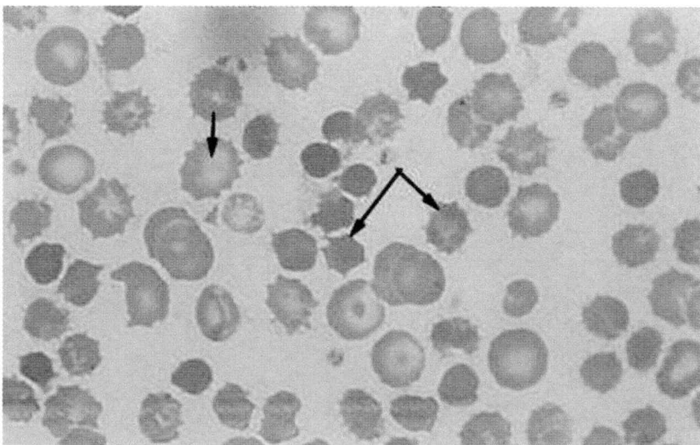

Q The treatment likely to be most effective in correcting this anemia includes:

A Erythropoietin 40,000 IU/week
B Oral prednisone 1 mg/kg/day
C Plasmapheresis—1.5 plasma volumes using albumin and saline replacement
D Liver transplantation
E Rituximab 375 mg/m^2 weekly for 4 weeks

Question 7

A 34-year-old woman is referred from a community free clinic for evaluation of leukocytosis. She is a poor historian and her speech is somewhat tangential. She admits to a past history of hospitalizations for psychiatric and medical problems; however, she does not know the nature of her illness nor does she know the names of the medications she takes. She admits to smoking and occasional use of alcohol. She denies fever or weight loss. Examination is unremarkable except for a disheveled appearance. Hematologic data are as follows:

Hematocrit:	33%
Hemoglobin	11 g/dL
Mean cell volume	78 fL
Platelet count	200,000/μL
Leukocyte count	12,800/μL
White cell differential	10,100/μL neutrophils
	2000/μL lymphocytes
	400/μL monocytes
	300/μL eosinophils

Q Which of the following is the most likely etiology of this patient's leukocytosis?

A Imipramine
B Chronic myeloid leukemia
C Lithium carbonate
D Chronic alcohol abuse
E Clozapine

Question 8

A 65-year-old woman presents to your clinic for evaluation of anemia and thrombocytopenia. She was found by her primary care doctor to have a hemoglobin of 9.8 g/dL and a platelet count of 105,000/μL, a normal white count and a mild increase in the peripheral blood monocytes. These cytopenias have progressed steadily over the past year, and therefore she was referred for evaluation. Her past medical history is significant for breast cancer 9 years ago. She received adjuvant chemotherapy at the time but cannot recall which drugs she was treated with. Your clinical suspicion is that this is likely myelodysplastic syndrome (MDS).

Q Which of the diagnostic results will be found in this patient?

A Bone marrow biopsy results showing 10% cellularity
B Marrow cytogenetics with a monosomy 7 abnormality
C 4+ fibrosis in the core biopsy
D Marrow cytogenetics showing the presence of the t(9;22)

Question 9

A 40-year-old man presents with epistaxis and is found to have multiple ecchymoses. His CBC reveals profound pancytopenia, and the peripheral blood and bone marrow confirm the diagnosis of acute myeloid leukemia.

Q Which of the following is the most appropriate induction chemotherapy for this patient?

A Daunorubicin 30 mg/m^2/day for 3 days, plus cytarabine 100 mg/m^2/day for 7 days by continuous infusion
B Daunorubicin 90 mg/m^2/day for 3 days, plus cytarabine 100 mg/m^2/day for 7 days by continuous infusion
C Daunorubicin 45–60 mg/m^2/day for 3 days, and cytarabine 500 mg/m^2/day for 7 days by continuous infusion
D Daunorubicin 45–60 mg/m^2/day for 3 days, and cytarabine 3 g/m^2 twice daily on days 1, 3 and 5 of induction
E Daunorubicin 45–60 mg/m^2/day for 3 days, and cytarabine 100 mg/m^2/day for 7 days by continuous infusion

Question 10

A 4-month-old boy presents with irritability. Physical findings include hepatosplenomegaly, generalized adenopathy, petechiae and pallor. His laboratory findings include hemoglobin 6 g/dL, WBC 47,000/μL (80% blasts) and platelets 37,000/μL. Bone marrow is replaced by blasts that are CD19$^+$, CD10$^-$.

Q Which of the following is the most likely chromosomal abnormality in this patient?

A t(1;19)
B t(9;22)
C t(4;11)
D t(12;21)
E Hypodiploidy

Question 11

A 67-year-old woman is referred for evaluation of an elevated white blood cell count, identified on a routine annual medical evaluation. She is asymptomatic. Examination shows no adenopathy or splenomegaly. CBC reveals WBC 29,000/μL with 82% lymphocytes, hemoglobin 13 g/dL and platelets 174,000/μL. The blood smear confirms increased small lymphocytes with occasional smudge cells. Flow cytometry of the peripheral blood lymphocytes is positive for kappa light chains, CD19, CD20 and CD23 but negative for CD3, CD38, FMC7 and ZAP-70. Fluorescence *in situ* hybridization (FISH) analysis reveals a chromosome 13q deletion.

Q Which of the following is the likely prognosis for this patient?

A An indolent course with median time to therapy >60 months
B An intermediate course with therapy likely within 36 months
C An aggressive course with therapy likely within 6–12 months
D Transformation to large cell lymphoma within 2–3 years
E Transformation to prolymphocytic leukemia within 2–3 years

Question 12

A 24-year-old woman was recently diagnosed with M1 AML with normal cytogenetics. She is undergoing induction chemotherapy with cytarabine and daunorubicin. She and her two siblings have been typed with the following results:

Patient A1,24; B18, 51; Cw7, 15; DRB1 11011, 04011
Brother A1,25; B18, 51; Cw7, 15; DRB1 11011, 04011
Sister A2,25; B51, 44; Cw16, 7; DRB1 15xx, 11xx

Q Which of the following would be the most effective form of transplantation for this patient?

A Allogeneic SCT—using her sister as the donor
B Allogeneic SCT—using her brother as the donor
C Autologous SCT
D Allogeneic SCT—using an HLA-identical unrelated donor

Question 13

A 27-year-old Caucasian woman is referred for management of idiopathic thrombocytopenic purpura (ITP) that has not responded to splenectomy. She was initially diagnosed by her gynecologist 4 months ago at the time of a routine examination. She had described some increase in menstrual bleeding and the gynecologist had noticed several petechiae on her feet and ankles and so ordered a CBC. The platelet count was 22,000/μL; the remainder of the CBC was normal. The patient was then evaluated by a hematologist; the diagnosis of ITP was established and prednisone, 1 mg/kg/day, was begun. After 3 months, a splenectomy was performed because the patient's platelet count fell to 20,000–30,000/μL each time the prednisone was tapered. Now, 1 month after splenectomy, she remains on prednisone, 20 mg/day, and her platelet count is 21,000/μL. Her hematologist has recommended treatment with rituximab, but she is reluctant to consider further treatment and only wants to stop prednisone.

At this time she has only the symptoms and signs of steroid toxicity. She has never had epistaxis or gingival bleeding; her menstrual bleeding is normal on the oral contraceptive pill; she has no petechiae but she does have purpura on her forearms, probably caused by the steroids.

Q What is the most appropriate management for this patient?

A Taper prednisone to 5 mg and 10 mg on alternate days and continue this regimen
B Taper and discontinue prednisone; treat with rituximab, 375 mg/m^2/week for 4 weeks
C Taper and discontinue prednisone; begin danazol, 200 mg four times daily
D Evaluate for the presence of an accessory spleen
E Taper and discontinue prednisone

Question 14

A 64-year-old, group O, Rh-positive male received 12 units of group O, Rh-positive packed red cells during repeat mitral valve replacement with a porcine valve 20 years after his first valve replacement. He has no comorbid conditions. Preoperative evaluation included a normal CBC and negative antibody screen. He became jaundiced 2 days after surgery with elevated liver enzymes and a total bilirubin of 20.7 mg/dL (direct fraction 7.0 mg/dL). His hemoglobin has dropped to 6.8 g/dL from the value of 11.0 g/dL obtained 2 h after the operation. No blood is noted in the stool or nasogastric tube drainage, and his chest tube drainage is minimal and serosanguinous.

Q Which test is most likely to reveal the cause of the postoperative anemia?

A Repeat antibody screen of the original sample
B Repeat ABO typing of the patient
C Repeat antibody screen of a new sample
D Repeat ABO typing of the transfused units

Question 15

A 58-year-old male is referred because of an elevated prothrombin time and activated partial thromboplastin time (APTT) from his dermatologist who wants to perform a skin biopsy. The patient denies any excessive bruising or bleeding in childhood or as an adult, although in recent months he has noted blood on the toilet tissue after bowel movements and increased bruising on his extremities. There is no family history of a bleeding disorder. Examination shows a scaly rash on his face and chest and several 4 × 5-cm ecchymoses on his lower extremities. Laboratory data are as follows:

Prothrombin time	18.4 s (normal 11.2–14.5 s)
1 : 1 mixing study	Corrected—13.6 s
APTT	47.5 s (normal 25.4–34.5 s)
1 : 1 mixing study	Not corrected—42.2 s immediate; 43.1 s at 1 h
Thrombin time	16.3 s (normal 14.8–24.6 s)
Fibrinogen	365 mg/dL

Q Which of the following tests would most likely diagnose the cause of this patient's condition?

A Lupus anticoagulant
B Factor VIII and factor VIII inhibitor assay
C Factors V and X
D Factors V, X and II
E Factor II and lupus anticoagulant

Question 16

A 45-year-old man consulted a second hematologist about treatment options. For the past 2 years, he has been under the care of his first hematologist for progressive stage IV follicular lymphoma, grade I. Recently, the first hematologist reviewed his treatment options. The patient was satisfied with the care he received from the first hematologist, but his family requested a second opinion. The second hematologist concurred with the first hematologist's diagnosis and discussed treatment options with the patient. He added allogeneic stem cell transplant to the list provided by the first hematologist. He then dictated a letter entitled 'Second Opinion' to the first hematologist with a copy to the primary physician. He began the section subtitled Treatment Options with the statement, 'I concur with the management and recommendations the patient has received.' Two days later, the second hematologist received an angry call from the first hematologist: the patient had complained that his treatment had been inappropriate. He stated that he had been told that he should have been referred for an allogeneic stem cell transplant.

Q Which of the following should the second hematologist have done to improve communication?

A Call the first hematologist at the time of consultation
B Videotape the encounter
C Send an e-mail to the first hematologist, the patient and the primary physician
D Call the patient the day after the visit

Question 17

Q Which of the following is the most sensitive test to detect relapse in a patient with CML after allogeneic stem cell transplant?

A Quantitative PCR of peripheral blood for t(9;22)
B Cytogenetic studies of bone marrow for t(9;22)
C FISH studies of bone marrow for t(9;22)
D Flow cytometric analysis of peripheral blood for leukemia markers

Question 18

A 43-year-old Russian immigrant complains of headaches. He is an automobile mechanic and he smokes two packs of cigarettes daily. He uses acetaminophen for pain but no other medications. His weight is 120 kg (body mass index 36 kg/m^2), blood pressure is 174/100 mmHg and transcutaneous oxygen saturation is 94% while breathing room air. He is plethoric and the spleen tip is palpable on abdominal examination. Laboratory data are as follows:

Hematocrit:	58%
Hemoglobin	19 g/dL
Mean cell volume	93 fL
Platelet count	530,000/μL
Leukocyte count	7200/μL
Serum creatinine	1.2 mg/dL
Serum erythropoietin level	2 mU/mL (normal: 2–20 mU/mL with normal hemoglobin)

Q Which of the following is the most likely cause of erythrocytosis in this patient?

A Gaisböck syndrome
B Hypoventilation syndrome
C Chuvash-type polycythemia
D Carbon monoxide poisoning
E Polycythemia vera

Question 19

A 20-year-old male complains of fatigue and increased shortness of breath on exertion. On examination, he appears to be a normal well-developed male although his thumbs appear underdeveloped and patches of hyperpigmentation are noted on his trunk. A CBC reveals severe pancytopenia. He does not report any toxic exposures. He has two siblings, one of whom 'was deformed at birth' and died in his late teens of leukemia. A bone marrow biopsy reveals cellularity of <10%; the bone marrow aspirate was characterized by hypocellular spicules with mostly residual plasma cells and lymphocytes. No abnormal cells were noted. Cytogenetic studies are pending.

Q What is the most likely laboratory test result that will confirm the diagnosis?

A Increased percentage of cells with aberrations on diepoxybutane (DEB) culture of peripheral blood mononuclear cells
B Decreased number of cells at G2M on flow cytometric analysis of bone marrow mononuclear cells for cell cycle distribution
C Increased percentage of cells with aberrations on DEB culture of fresh bone marrow mononuclear cells
D Increased percentage of myeloblasts on myeloperoxidase stain of bone marrow aspirate smear

Question 20

A 72-year-old man with a 3-year history of myelodysplasia presents to your clinic for his routine follow-up appointment.

Over the past 2 weeks he has had brief episodes of chest heaviness while walking up a hill. On examination, his stool hemoccult test is negative. His CBC shows WBC 5400/μL, HCT 24%, platelets 96,000/μL. His corrected reticulocyte count is 1%.

Q The most appropriate acute therapy for this patient is:

A Start epoetin alfa once weekly
B Start darbepoetin alfa once every 2 weeks
C Transfuse 2 IU packed red blood cells (PRBC)
D Start prednisone 60 mg/day orally
E Start epoetin alfa once weekly and filgrastim daily

Question 21

A 49-year-old woman has been having heavy menstrual periods as she nears menopause. She is noted to be anemic with a hemoglobin of 7.0 g/dL, an MCV of 69 fL and a ferritin of 1 ng/mL. The patient weighs 68 kg (150 lb) and has absent iron stores.

Q What is the total amount of supplemental iron that would be needed to correct her hemoglobin to 12 g/dL and replenish her iron stores?

A 510 mg
B 730 mg
C 1050 mg
D 1350 mg
E 1490 mg

Question 22

A 16-year-old boy has been anemic and jaundiced since the age of 6 years. On examination, he has mild splenomegaly. He has a lactic dehydrogenase (LDH) of 630 U/L, but a relatively low reticulocyte count of 0.3%. His ferritin is markedly increased with an increased iron and increased transferrin saturation. His Coombs test is negative. His peripheral smear is significant for anisopoikilocytosis and macrocytosis. Review of his marrow reveals multinucleated erythroblasts. His anemia and jaundice have become more severe, to the point where he may need red cell transfusions.

Q Which of the following treatments is most likely to resolve his anemia and jaundice?

A Iron chelation therapy
B Splenectomy
C Erythropoietin
D Intravenous immunoglobulin
E Prednisone

Question 23

A 4-year-old Caucasian boy has been brought to the endoscopy suite for removal of a bezoar. Prior to the procedure he is administered benzocaine spray to anesthetize the oropharynx. Within 30 min the patient becomes visibly cyanotic, restless and tachycardic. He remains hemodynamically stable. His oxygen saturation by pulse oximetry is 73%, and on the arterial blood gas Pao_2 is 95 mmHg. His blood sample is described as appearing dark brown. He is placed on 100% oxygen via facemask. His prior history is unremarkable, and there is no history of other drug exposure.

Q What is the most appropriate management for this patient's condition?

A No further intervention
B Red blood cell exchange
C Methylene blue 1 mg/kg over 5 min intravenously
D Methylprednisolone sodium succinate (Solu-medrol) 125 mg intravenously
E Immediate hyperbaric oxygen

Question 24

A 42-year-old woman was recently diagnosed with polycythemia vera (PV) after presenting with aquagenic pruritus, headaches and painful burning in the fingers and toes. Her past medical history is notable for a lower extremity deep venous thrombosis while on oral contraceptives 5 years ago. She is now 8 weeks pregnant. Physical examination discloses a thin woman with a palpable spleen tip and patches of skin erythema on two toes with superficial ulcerations. She has been started on weekly phlebotomies and aspirin, 100 mg/day. Hematologic data are as follows:

Hematocrit	49%
Hemoglobin	16.4 g/dL
Leukocyte count	6800/μL
Platelet count	500,000/μL
Peripheral smear	Mild erythrocyte anisocytosis, normal leukocytes, large and giant platelets

Q Which of the following is the most appropriate additional management for this patient?

A Interferon-α
B Low-molecular-weight heparin
C Hydroxyurea
D Anagrelide
E No additional treatment

Question 25

A 58-year-old man is admitted to the hospital with fever, cellulitis and severe neutropenia. His past medical history is notable for hypercholesterolemia, diet-controlled diabetes and inflammatory arthritis. Current medications include naproxen, glucosamine and simvastatin. Examination reveals painful erythema extending from the dorsum of the right foot to the ankle. Multiple joint deformities are found in the hands. There is no lymphadenopathy but the spleen is palpated 5 cm below the left costal margin. Hematologic data are as follows:

Hematocrit	40%
Hemoglobin	13.8 g/dL
Mean cell volume	93 fL
Platelet count	200,000/μL
Leukocyte count	5900/μL
White cell differential	80/μL neutrophils 5220/μL lymphocytes 300/μL monocytes 300/μL eosinophils

Q Which of the following tests will be most helpful in identifying the cause of this patient's neutropenia?

A Peripheral blood assay for T-cell receptor gene rearrangement
B Rheumatoid factor assay
C Marrow morphology assessment and cytogenetics
D Immunophenotypic analysis of blood and/or marrow cells
E Peripheral blood assay for B-cell immunoglobulin gene rearrangement

Question 26

A 52-year-old man develops an acute ischemic left hemispheric cerebrovascular accident 2 days after elective shoulder surgery. His past medical history is remarkable only for a sports-related femur fracture and arthroscopic knee surgery 7 years ago, neither of which were associated with any sequelae. He has no history of diabetes, hypercholesterolemia or smoking. Physical examination is notable for aphasia and right hemiparesis. The surgical wound is dry but mildly swollen. Splenomegaly is palpable 3 cm below the left costal margin. Duplex ultrasound studies of the lower extremities and of the carotid arteries found no evidence of thrombosis or occlusion. Echocardiogram found no evidence of valvular vegetation or right-to-left intracardiac shunt. Postoperative hematology data are as follows:

Hematocrit	53%
MCV	93 fL
Leukocyte count	9800/μL
Platelet count	690,000/μL
Peripheral blood smear	Mild red cell anisocytosis, occasional basophils, increased platelets and a rare giant platelet

Preoperative hematology data were as follows:

Hematocrit	57%
Hemoglobin	18.9 g/dL
Leukocyte count	7600/μL
Platelet count	550,000/μL

Q Which of the following is the most likely cause of this patient's thromboembolic complication?

A Postoperative immobilization
B Elevated blood viscosity
C Factor V Leiden mutation
D Disseminated intravascular coagulopathy (DIC)
E Surgery-induced hypercoagulability

Question 27

A 65-year-old man with a known history of MDS has been a patient of yours for the past 2 years. More recently, he has had a gradual decrease in his hemoglobin to 8.0 g/dL as well as a steadily decreasing platelet count, which is now at 45,000/μL. A repeat bone marrow biopsy was obtained which showed a hypercellular marrow with 25% myeloblasts. He had only 4% myeloblasts approximately 2 years earlier.

Q Which of the following statements is correct?

A There is an 80% chance of achieving a complete remission of the disease with induction chemotherapy
B Cytogenetic results obtained after induction therapy are likely to show a complete cytogenetic remission

C The risk of relapse of his AML is the same as that of a patient with *de novo* AML undergoing the same chemotherapy regimen
D Cytogenetic studies on the most recent bone marrow aspirate are likely to reveal new cytogenetic abnormalities not present on the previous sample

Question 28

A 25-year-old man presents to the emergency room with epistaxis, melena and dyspnea on exertion. His examination shows multiple ecchymoses on the lower extremities. His laboratory data show a white blood cell count of 1200/μL, hemoglobin of 6.6 g/dL and a platelet count of 11,000/μL. The white blood cell count differential on the peripheral blood shows that approximately 80% of the cells are blasts. His serum fibrinogen is 72 mg/dL, prothrombin time (PT) is prolonged at 28.5 s, and partial thromboplastin time (PTT) is prolonged at 50 s. A bone marrow biopsy is performed and the diagnosis of acute promyelocytic leukemia is established.

Q Which of the following is the most appropriate induction therapy for this patient?

A Daunorubicin 60 mg/m^2/day for 3 days, and cytarabine 100 mg/m^2/day for 7 days by continuous infusion
B Daunorubicin 90 mg/m^2/day for 3 days, plus all-*trans* retinoic acid (ATRA)
C Idarubicin 12 mg/m^2/day for 4 days, plus ATRA, plus arsenic trioxide 10 mg/m^2/day for 25 days
D ATRA, plus arsenic trioxide 10 mg/m^2/day for 25 days
E Daunorubicin 60 mg/m^2/day for 3 days, plus ATRA

Question 29

A 4-year-old girl presents with fevers and bone pains. There is no organomegaly or adenopathy. Laboratory data include hemoglobin 8.5 g/dL, WBC 6000/μL (1% blasts) and platelets 85,000/μL. Her bone marrow is replaced with blasts that are CD19$^+$, CD10$^+$.

Q Which of the following would be the most favorable chromosomal finding in childhood ALL?

A Hyperdiploidy
B Hypodiploidy
C t(9;22)
D t(4;11)
E Triploidy for chromosomes 4, 10 and 17

Question 30

A 74-year-old man has progressing B-CLL treated with oral chlorambucil plus prednisone. After 3 months of therapy his WBC has decreased from 140,000 to 60,000/μL but his adenopathy and splenomegaly have worsened and his hemoglobin has decreased from 11.9 to 10.5 g/dL. LDH and chemistries are normal. He has had no fever or night sweats but is fatigued.

Q Which of the following would be indicated in this patient?

A Cyclophosphamide
B Fludarabine
C Alemtuzumab
D Rituximab

Question 31

Q Which would be the optimal stem cell source to minimize the risk of graft-versus-host disease in an adult?

A HLA-identical cord blood
B HLA-identical mobilized peripheral blood stem cells
C HLA-identical elutriated lymphocyte-depleted bone marrow
D HLA-identical unrelated donor peripheral blood stem cells

Question 32

A 27-year-old woman is referred for evaluation of thrombocytopenia, which was discovered incidentally during an evaluation for employment. She is healthy and takes no medications. She plays on a soccer team, and has noticed some bruises, but considered them to be normal. She has noticed no petechiae, no increased menstrual bleeding and no other bleeding symptoms. Otherwise, findings on the history and physical examination are normal. The CBC results are normal, except for a platelet count of 42,000/μL. The blood chemistry profile is normal and urinalysis is normal. Examination of the peripheral blood smear is normal except for the moderate thrombocytopenia.

Q What is the most appropriate management for this patient?

A Repeat CBC in 1 month
B Reassure her and discharge her without plans for additional platelet counts

C Therapy with prednisone, 1 mg/kg/day
D Bone marrow aspiration and biopsy
E CT scan of the chest and abdomen

Question 33

Fifteen minutes after starting a transfusion of group A, Rh-negative packed red cells, a patient typed as group A, Rh-positive has new-onset fever, back pain, abdominal cramping, rigors and dyspnea. Hypotension is also noted. Red urine is evident in the Foley catheter bag, but urine output decreases in the next hour. The pretransfusion antibody screen was negative.

Q What is the most likely cause of this patient's symptoms?

A Transfusion of Rh-negative blood
B Laboratory errors in compatibility testing
C Bacterial contamination of the unit
D Mislabeling of the pretransfusion sample
E Cytokines elaborated by donor white cells

Question 34

A 13-year-old female presents with menorrhagia. She has experienced six menstrual periods and states that each period lasts 8–10 days and requires a change of pads or tampons every 2–3 h during days 2 and 3. A recent CBC by her family practitioner shows that her hemoglobin is 10.9 g/dL and her MCV is 79 pg/mL. She had epistaxis as a younger child, but the bleeding was not severe enough to require medical attention. Her mother has a history of heavy menstrual periods and a maternal aunt had bleeding after delivery of a full-term infant for which she received red cells. Examination does not show ecchymoses or petechiae or other signs of bleeding. Laboratory data are as follows:

Prothrombin time	13.9 s (normal 11.2–14.5 s)
APTT	34.9 s (normal 25.4–34.5 s)
Thrombin time	20.4 s (normal 14.8–24.6 s)
Fibrinogen	298 mg/dL

Q Which of the following tests should be ordered in the evaluation of this patient?

A Bleeding time
B Platelet aggregation studies
C von Willebrand factor levels (activity and antigen) and factor VIII
D Electron microscopy of the patient's platelets

Question 35

You are asked to provide recommendations for prophylaxis of deep vein thrombosis (DVT) in an otherwise healthy 76-year-old man who is scheduled for a right total knee replacement. Five years ago he had a left total hip replacement without prophylaxis. Two weeks after the surgery he suffered a symptomatic left lower extremity DVT for which he was treated with warfarin for 3 months. He has no other history of thromboembolic disease. His family history is negative for thrombophilia.

Q Which of the following is the most appropriate next step in the evaluation and management of this patient's risk for deep venous thrombosis?

A Evaluation for thrombophilia
B Low-dose aspirin and dextran the day before surgery and then daily until discharge
C Postoperative low-molecular-weight heparin (LMWH)
D Graded compression stockings and early ambulation

Question 36

Q Which of the following is the most appropriate response to a positive RT-PCR for the t(9;22) in a patient who achieves molecular remission after stem cell transplantation?

A The study should be repeated
B The patient should be reinduced with high-dose chemotherapy
C Donor lymphocyte infusion should be recommended immediately
D The patient should be treated with imatinib

Question 37

A 30-year-old male complains of fatigue and increased shortness of breath on exertion. On examination, he appears to be a normal well-developed male although his thumbs appear underdeveloped and patches of hyperpigmentation are noted on his trunk. A CBC reveals severe pancytopenia. He does not report any toxic exposures. He has two siblings, one of whom 'was deformed at birth' and died in his late teens of leukemia. A bone marrow biopsy reveals cellularity of <10%; the bone marrow aspirate was characterized by hypocellular spicules with mostly residual plasma cells and lymphocytes. No abnormal cells were noted. Diepoxybutane

(DEB) culture of peripheral blood mononuclear cells reveals an increased percentage of cells with aberrations.

Cytogenetic analysis of the bone marrow sample revealed a normal karyotype in 20 out of 20 metaphases. His remaining sibling is HLA typed and noted to be a complete match and is tested and confirmed not to have the same abnormality as the patient.

Q Which of the following is the most appropriate treatment option?

A Immunosuppression with antithymocyte globulin 40 mg/kg for 4 days and cyclosporine 12 mg/kg/day
B Matched sibling allogeneic stem cell transplant with total body irradiation of 1000 cGy with lung shielding + cyclophosphamide 60 mg/kg/day intravenously for 2 days as conditioning
C Induction chemotherapy with idarubicin 12 mg/day for 3 days and cytosine arabinoside at 100 mg/m^2 for 7 days.
D Matched sibling allogeneic stem cell transplant with total body irradiation of 500 cGy with lung shielding + cyclophosphamide 20 mg/kg intravenously for 2 days as conditioning

Question 38

A 45-year-old man presents for his third cycle of CHOP-rituximab therapy for stage III large B-cell lymphoma. His cervical adenopathy has markedly decreased in size since the beginning of chemotherapy. Although he feels well, he complains of fatigue. His CBC shows WBC 3500/μL, HCT 27% and platelets 317,000/μL.

Q What is the most appropriate therapy for this patient's fatigue?

A No intervention
B Transfuse 2 IU of PRBC today.
C Initiation of therapy with epoetin alfa once every 3 weeks
D Initiation of therapy with darbepoetin alfa once every 3 weeks

Question 39

A 27-year-old man with type 1a glycogen storage disease is found to have microcytic anemia that is refractory to oral iron supplementation and slow to respond to intravenous iron dextran. His laboratory studies are significant for iron of 70 μg/dL, a total iron-binding capacity (TIBC) of 210 μg/dL and a serum ferritin of 560 ng/mL. The patient is found to have large hepatic adenomas and undergoes resection. His anemia subsequently resolves.

Q Which protein is most likely responsible for his anemia?

A Hepcidin
B HFE
C Divalent metal transporter 1 (DMT1)
D Ceruloplasmin
E Hephestin

Question 40

A 62-year-old female hemodialysis patient with angiodysplasia requires intravenous iron dextran in addition to erythropoietin to maintain a hemoglobin of 11 g/dL. She has become progressively intolerant to iron dextran and recently had an anaphylactic reaction characterized by hypotension, pruritus, nausea and vomiting.

Q Which iron preparation would be best to replace her iron stores and maintain erythropoiesis?

A Oral ferrous sulfate
B Oral ferrous gluconate
C Intravenous iron dextran preceded by hydroxyzine
D Intravenous iron dextran preceded by prednisone
E Intravenous iron sucrose

Question 41

A 45-year-old man was treated 3 years ago for aplastic anemia. He responded well to treatment with antithymocyte globulin (ATG) and cyclosporine with normalization of his blood counts. He subsequently was lost to follow-up until recently when he was noted to have mild pancytopenia with an absolute neutrophil count (ANC) of 1200/μL, HCT 32% and platelet count of 123,000/μL. For the past 3 days he has complained of significant right upper quadrant pain. Hepatic vein occlusion is subsequently diagnosed by Doppler ultrasound. Anticoagulant therapy with heparin is administered and the patient clinically improves. Prior personal and family history is negative for any thrombotic disorders.

Q Which of the following tests is the most likely to lead to the proper diagnosis?

A Flow cytometry of peripheral blood leukocytes for CD59
B PCR analysis for factor V Leiden

C Analysis of burst-forming units of bone marrow red blood cell precursors (BFU-E)
D Vitamin B_{12} level

Question 42

A 33-year-old man is referred for further evaluation of intra-abdominal lymphadenopathy, mild splenomegaly and leukocytosis. These abnormalities were discovered during a recent work-up for chronic recurrent abdominal pain and episodic fever. He is originally from Turkey but has lived in the USA for 3 years. He drinks two beers daily and takes antacids and acetaminophen with codeine. He reports a 25-year history of sporadic unprovoked episodes of fever and pain in the abdomen and joints that last for 1–3 days. A recent CT scan of the abdomen revealed a small amount of peritoneal fluid, a homogeneously enlarged spleen, at 12 cm longitudinal length, and scattered 1–1.5-cm mesenteric lymph nodes. Blood chemistries and liver function tests were normal except for a creatinine of 1.3 mg/dL. Urinalysis revealed 4+ protein without red blood cells, white cells or casts. On examination, the patient is afebrile, thin and nonicteric. Palpation of the abdomen elicits diffuse mild tenderness and voluntary guarding but without rebound tenderness. No peripheral lymphadenopathy or palpable hepatosplenomegaly are appreciated. There is a small effusion in the left knee joint. Hematologic data are as follows:

Hematocrit:	48%
Hemoglobin	15.9 g/dL
Platelet count	290,000/μL
Leukocyte count	15,500/μL
White cell differential	11,400/μL neutrophils
	3100/μL lymphocytes
	700/μL monocytes
	300/μL eosinophils

Q Which of the following abnormalities will most likely be discovered with additional studies?

A Urate crystals on joint aspiration and *BCR-ABL* gene rearrangement in peripheral blood leukocytes
B Amyloidosis on renal biopsy and *MEFV* gene mutations in peripheral blood leukocytes
C Mast cells on lymph node biopsy and an Asp-816-Val c-*kit* point mutation
D Hemophagocytic histiocytes on lymph node biopsy and *PRF1* gene mutations in peripheral blood leukocytes
E Small cleaved lymphoma cells on lymph node biopsy and *IgH-BCL2* gene rearrangement

Question 43

A 75-year-old woman with a new diagnosis of MDS comes to your office for consultation. She is only mildly anemic with a platelet count of 550,000/μL. Her bone marrow biopsy showed <5% blasts. Cytogenetic studies showed 5q- as the only cytogenetic abnormality.

Q Which of the following is the most appropriate next step in the management of this patient?

A Given her age and bone marrow findings, consideration should be given to proceeding with a nonmyeloablative transplant
B She should be followed closely in the outpatient clinic with no therapy initially
C Intensive chemotherapy approaches should be considered to prevent imminent progression of her disease to AML
D Given the thrombocytosis, she should be started on anagrelide therapy to control the thrombocytosis

Question 44

Q Which of the following is most consistent following G-CSF or GM-CSF during induction therapy in patients with AML?

A Improvement in the complete remission rate
B Reduction in the duration of neutropenia
C Reduction in induction mortality
D Improvement in overall survival

Question 45

A 54-year-old woman is referred for evaluation of night sweats and weight loss over the past 2 months. She has been unable to continue her work as a school teacher for the preceding 3 weeks because of fatigue and chest discomfort. Examination reveals a thin, ill-appearing woman with no palpable adenopathy or splenomegaly. Chest X-ray demonstrates an anterior mediastinal mass; chest CT scan confirms a 5-cm mass plus enlarged pericardial nodes. Abdominal and pelvic CTs show multiple 2–3-cm para-aortic nodes, marrow biopsy is normal and PET scan shows uptake only at the known sites identified by CT. A CT-guided core biopsy reveals diffuse large B-cell lymphoma. She is mildly anemic, and LDH is normal. Treatment with R-CHOP (cyclophosphamide, doxorubicin, vincristine, prednisone, rituximab) is initiated, with prompt resolution of B symptoms after one cycle.

Q Her prognosis for 5-year survival with 6–8 cycles of induction therapy is approximately:

A 90%
B 70%
C 50%
D 30%
E <15%

Question 46

A 63-year-old man was originally diagnosed with stage IVB follicular (grade 2) lymphoma 6 years ago. He had pancytopenia resulting from marrow involvement and was given CVP for eight cycles. He achieved a complete remission. Four years later, he developed recurrent disease and a biopsy demonstrated persistent follicular lymphoma. He was given CVP for eight cycles and again achieved a partial remission. One year later, he developed a histologic transformation to diffuse large cell lymphoma. At that time, he was given ESHAP for four cycles and achieved a complete remission. He is now referred for evaluation of possible transplantation.

Q Which of the following is the most appropriate recommendation for this patient?

A No transplantation as he is in complete remission
B Autologous stem cell transplantation
C Myeloablative allogeneic stem cell transplantation
D Nonmyeloablative allogeneic stem cell transplantation

Question 47

An 8-year-old boy presents with bruising. He has hepatosplenomegaly, adenopathy and petechiae. Laboratory data include hemoglobin 8 g/dL, WBC 10,000/μL (2% blasts) and platelets 127,000/μL.

Q Which of the following is the most favorable prognostic factor in childhood ALL?

A Age 1–9 years with a WBC ≤50,000/μL
B Age >9 years or a WBC >50,000/μL
C Age <1 year
D T-cell ALL
E t(9;22)

Question 48

A 78-year-old female with relapsed chronic lymphocytic leukemia was given leukocyte-reduced packed red cells and platelet concentrates for intravenous catheter placement before her third cycle of fludarabine therapy. Two weeks later she developed an erythematous indurated rash on her trunk and extremities, jaundice, elevated transaminases and watery diarrhea. A CBC revealed pancytopenia with an absolute reticulocyte count of 15,000/μL.

Q What is the most likely cause of these new findings?

A Autoimmune pancytopenia
B Systemic CMV reactivation
C Fludarabine toxicity
D Graft-versus-host disease
E Richter transformation

Question 49

A 6-year-old male is hospitalized because of excessive bleeding after a thumb laceration. He has a history of spontaneous bruising and frequent epistaxis since age 2 years. There is no family history of a bleeding disorder. Examination shows five 4-cm ecchymoses on both lower extremities and a lacerated thumb. Laboratory data are as follows:

Prothrombin time	13.6 s (normal 11.2–14.5 s)
APTT	29.9 s (normal 25.4–34.5 s)
Thrombin time	18.4 s (normal 14.8–24.6 s)
Fibrinogen	285 mg/dL
Platelet count	344,000/mL
von Willebrand factor assays	Normal
Platelet function analyzer	Normal closure times

Q What other test will be most helpful in the diagnosis of this patient?

A Platelet aggregation studies
B Immunologic fibrinogen level
C α_2-Antiplasmin level
D Factor XII level
E Examination of the peripheral smear

Question 50

You are asked to evaluate the risk of bleeding in a 56-year-old Swedish-American woman who plans to donate a kidney to her daughter. She denies any current bleeding problems. At age 47, symptoms of endometriosis prompted a hysterectomy. The procedure was complicated by postoperative bleeding which led to surgical re-exploration and transfusion with 6 units of packed red blood cells. A hematologic evaluation was never performed. Prior to the hysterectomy, menstrual blood flow was said to be heavy. Her mother was diagnosed by a hematologist as a 'bleeder', but further details are not available. Her physical examination is normal except for an abdominal scar, and her platelet count, INR and APTT are normal.

Q Which of the following is the most appropriate step in the evaluation of this patient?

A Perform a bleeding time and measure factor XI
B Measure von Willebrand factor antigen and factor VIII and perform a ristocetin cofactor assay
C Proceed with the operation without further preoperative hemostatic evaluation
D Measure fibrinogen using an immunologic method

Question 51

A 24-year-old woman develops a deep venous thrombosis. The test for resistance to activated protein C (APC) is abnormal.

Q Which of the following should be carried out next to further evaluate this patient?

A Southern blot of genomic DNA prepared from peripheral blood, digested with MnlI and probed with a fragment of the protein C gene
B RT-PCR amplification of peripheral blood using factor V-specific primers
C PCR amplification of peripheral blood using factor V-specific primers followed by MnlI digestion of the PCR product
D Linkage analysis of the patient, her siblings and parents using restriction fragment length polymorphisms (RFLPs)

Question 52

A 16-year-old girl is referred for the evaluation of thrombocytopenia. She has a history of learning difficulties. Physical examination reveals short stature (<third percentile) without other musculoskeletal abnormalities. Her hemoglobin is 11.4 g/dL, white blood cell count 3.9×10^9/L with absolute neutrophil count 1.9×10^9/L, platelets 18×10^9/L and hemoglobin F percentage 15%. Bone marrow examination reveals hypocellular trilineage myelodysplasia and 8% blasts. Karyotypic analysis reveals trisomy 8 in 4 of 20 metaphases.

Q Which of the following is the most likely diagnosis?

A Dyskeratosis congenita
B Schwachman–Diamond syndrome
C Amegakaryocytic thrombocytopenia
D Fanconi anemia

Question 53

Q Which of the following statements about the use of filgrastim (granulocyte colony-stimulating factor [G-CSF]) therapy in peripheral blood stem cell transplantation is true?

A It improves mortality
B It reduces the incidence of infectious episodes following stem cell mobilization with high-dose cyclophosphamide
C It increases the incidence of acute graft-versus-host disease
D It causes headache, bone pain and fatigue in most patients

Question 54

A healthy 28-year-old female was diagnosed with homozygous hereditary hemochromatosis (C282Y/C282Y) through genetic screening after her alcoholic father was diagnosed with cirrhosis. The patient is asymptomatic, has normal menstrual periods and abstains from drinking alcohol. She has never had her iron studies checked prior to today's visit. She is concerned about what this diagnosis will mean to her both immediately and in the future. She is married to a healthy Caucasian male.

Current iron studies include the following:

Serum iron	120 μg/dL (normal, 42–135 μg/dL)
Serum total iron-binding capacity	300 μg/dL (normal, 225–430 μg/dL)
Transferrin saturation	39% (normal, 20–50%)
Ferritin	189 ng/mL (normal, 30–400 ng/mL)

Q Which of the following statements about this patient's prognosis and follow-up is true?

A She will likely develop clinical iron overload later in life
B All her offspring will be heterozygous for the C282Y mutation

C Phlebotomy should be initiated at the initiation of menopause
D Screening for hepatoma by ultrasound and alfa-fetoprotein should be performed annually
E Ferritin values should be monitored periodically throughout her life

Question 55

A 70-year-old woman with diabetes, hypertension and end-stage renal disease has recently been noted to have declining hemoglobin levels despite supplemental erythropoietin given at 100 U/kg three times weekly. Iron studies reveal an elevated ferritin of 650 μg/L, with corresponding increased serum iron of 250 μg/dL and iron saturation of 45%. She has normal folic acid and cobalamin levels.

Q Which of the following interventions will most likely improve her anemia?
A Begin iron chelation
B Substitute darbepoetin for erythropoietin
C Add intravenous ascorbic acid
D Supplement oral iron at 325 mg $FeSO_4$ three times daily
E Supplement iron dextran intravenously

Question 56

A 24-year-old African-American man is sent to you for evaluation of anemia. He remembers presenting to the emergency room a few times as a child for evaluation of pain in his legs. Otherwise his past history is entirely benign. Both of his parents are healthy. His mother is known to have an asymptomatic microcytic anemia and his father is known to have a normal hemoglobin and hematocrit. Laboratory data include the following:

WBC count	6700/μL	Hemoglobin electrophoresis
HCT	31%	S = 62%
MCV	73 fL	A = 25%
Platelet count	424,000/μL	A_2 = 4.8%
Reticulocyte count	3%	F = 8%
Iron studies	Normal	

The blood smear reveals hypochromia, microcytosis, poikilocytosis and target-shaped red blood cells. No sickle cells are seen.

Q Which of the following is the most likely diagnosis?
A Sickle cell trait
B S-β^+ thalassemia
C S-β° thalassemia
D Sickle cell anemia with hereditary persistence of fetal hemoglobin

Question 57

A 55-year-old Chinese-American woman is transferred to the intensive care unit with confusion, progressive pulmonary infiltrates and hypotension. She was admitted to the hospital the previous day for evaluation of fever, lymphadenopathy, malaise and mild pancytopenia. Blood and urine cultures are negative and the initial chest X-ray was clear. Additional studies are pending. She has a long history of systemic lupus erythematosus, recently controlled with hydroxychloroquine, azathioprine and low-dose prednisone. On examination, the patient is stuporous without focal or lateralizing neurologic deficits or meningismus. Skin and sclera are icteric with scattered ecchymoses on the distal upper extremities. Enlarged lymph nodes, measuring 1.5–3 cm, are found in the cervical, axillary, epitrochlear and inguinal regions. The liver and spleen extend 4 cm and 3 cm below the costal margins, respectively. Laboratory data are as follows:

Hematocrit	28%
Hemoglobin	9.8 g/dL
Platelet count	58,000/μL
Reticulocyte count	75,000/μL
Leukocyte count	2500/μL
White cell differential	1100/μL neutrophils 200/μL bands 700/μL lymphocytes 100/μL atypical lymphocytes 300/μL monocytes 100/μL eosinophils
Blood smear	Mild erythrocyte anisocytosis, decreased platelets with occasional bands and atypical lymphocytes; no schistocytes or blast forms seen
Prothrombin time/INR	13.4 s/1.2
Activated partial thromboplastin time	43 s
Fibrinogen	110 mg/dL
D-dimer	0.38 μg/mL
Bilirubin, total	3.8 mg/dL
Bilirubin, direct	2.9 mg/dL
Alanine aminotransferase	230 U/L
Aspartate aminotransferase	350 U/L
Alkaline phosphatase	220 U/L
Creatinine	1.9 mg/dL

Bone marrow aspiration reveals normal trilineage maturation with left-shifted myeloid precursors, occasional lymphocytes and plasma cells, and scattered cytophagocytic histiocytes (see Figure).

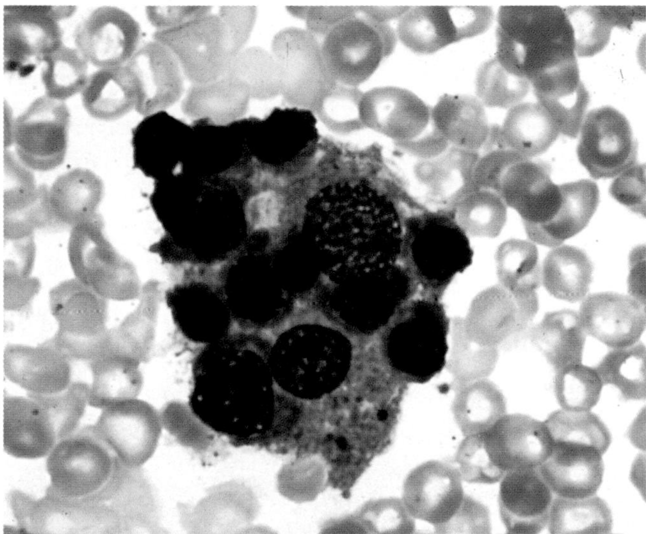

Q Which of the following interventions is most important for the appropriate initial management of this patient?

A High-dose cyclophosphamide administration
B Lymph node biopsy
C Plasma exchange
D Ganciclovir administration
E Open lung biopsy

Question 58

A 42-year-old man with recent-onset migraine headaches and infrequent epistaxis was referred for evaluation and recommendations regarding a platelet count of 950,000/μL. He takes acetaminophen for exercise-related musculoskeletal pain. Hematocrit is 37%, MCV is 90 fL and leukocyte count is 9800/μL. The patient weighs 120 kg. Hepatosplenomegaly cannot be accurately assessed by examination. Abdominal ultrasound reveals splenomegaly measuring 18 cm in longitudinal diameter.

Q Which of the following additional test results in this patient would confer the least favorable prognosis?

A Hypercellular marrow with stainable iron
B Hypercellular marrow with megakaryocyte clusters
C Giant platelets on blood smear
D Abnormal platelet aggregation
E Grade 2+ marrow reticulin fibrosis with leukoerythroblastosis on blood smear

Question 59

A 50-year-old man is referred to you by another hematologist for a second opinion. He initially presented with significant pancytopenias and has required transfusion support with both packed red cells and platelets. A bone marrow biopsy was obtained and showed marked hypocellularity at 15% with mild dysplastic changes seen in the erythroid cell line. The referring doctor is unclear as to how best to characterize this disorder and plan for treatment.

Q Which of the following tests and results would be most useful in making the diagnosis?

A Poor marrow progenitor growth in culture
B Normal platelet aggregation *in vitro*
C Cytogenetic studies from bone marrow showing monosomy 7
D Normal expression of CD55 and CD59

Question 60

A 26-year-old woman with AML and the t(8;21), but no other cytogenetic abnormality, achieves a complete remission after induction therapy with daunorubicin and cytarabine. The patient has two brothers, one of whom is HLA-identical with the patient.

Q Which one of the following would be the most appropriate post-remission strategy to prevent relapse?

A One cycle of consolidation chemotherapy with high-dose cytarabine, followed by a low-intensity matched related donor stem cell transplantation
B One cycle of consolidation chemotherapy with a repeat of her induction chemotherapy, followed by a low-intensity matched related donor stem cell transplantation
C Four cycles of consolidation chemotherapy with high-dose cytarabine
D Four cycles of consolidation with high-dose cytarabine, followed by an autologous stem cell transplant
E A fully ablative HLA-matched related stem cell transplant

Question 61

A 4-year-old girl presents with low-grade fevers and lethargy. Physical examination shows multiple small lymph nodes. There is no organomegaly. Laboratory data include hemoglobin 7.5 g/dL, WBC 4500/μL and platelets 35,000/μL. The bone marrow is replaced by $CD19^+$, $CD10^+$, TdT^+ lymphoblasts. The leukemia karyotype is 47XX, t(12;21). There are no blasts in the cerebrospinal fluid.

Q Which of the following would be indicated as central nervous system prophylaxis in this patient?

A Cranial irradiation plus intrathecal methotrexate
B Craniospinal irradiation
C Intrathecal methotrexate
D Intrathecal methotrexate, hydrocortisone and cytosine arabinoside

Question 62

A 56-year-old man receives six cycles of R-CHOP chemotherapy (cyclophosphamide, doxorubicin, vincristine, prednisone, rituximab) for stage III diffuse large B-cell lymphoma and achieves complete remission, with normal CT scans after cycle 4. Fourteen months later he develops fever and night sweats. Repeat CT shows a 6-cm retroperitoneal mass, and biopsy is positive for relapsed large B-cell lymphoma. Bone marrow biopsy is negative. ECOG performance status is 1. After two cycles of R-ICE chemotherapy (rituximab, ifosfamide, carboplatin, etoposide) he is again in complete remission by CT scan.

Q Which of the following would be indicated for additional therapy for this patient?

A Two additional cycles of R-ICE and follow-up CT scans at 4 months
B Autologous stem cell transplantation
C Allogeneic stem cell transplantation
D Scheduled rituximab maintenance therapy
E Radioimmunotherapy

Question 63

A 45-year-old man with AML is referred for consideration of transplantation. The patient at presentation of his AML was felt to have standard risk features. His treating hematologist and the patient decided to treat with chemotherapy, reserving transplant for relapse, should it occur. After induction he received consolidation with high-dose Ara-C. On a routine visit a year after his initial treatment, pancytopenia was noted, whereas his counts had been normal 2 weeks earlier. Bone marrow aspiration showed relapse of his AML with 70% blasts on differential. Unfortunately, the patient's relapse proved very difficult to treat, requiring several attempts at reinduction and gemtuzumab ozogamicin before entering a tenuous remission. At the direction of the nearest transplant center, HLA typing had been performed while the patient was being treated. Typing of the patient's siblings showed that one sister (para 3, CMV-positive) and one brother (CMV-negative) were HLA-identical and one other brother (CMV-negative) was haplo-identical. The patient was CMV-negative. The patient's wife was 3 months' pregnant. A preliminary search of the National Marrow Donor Program (NMDP) registry showed that there were eight potential matches, but none had high-resolution typing performed.

Q Who should serve as the donor?

A Wait for the baby to be born and collect the cord blood as the stem cell source
B Use the haplo-identical brother
C Complete high-resolution typing on the eight potential donors in the registry
D Use the HLA-identical sister
E Use the HLA-identical brother

Question 64

A 19-year-old previously healthy African-American woman had an uncomplicated first pregnancy with delivery of a healthy infant. Nine days following delivery she returned to her obstetrician with severe weakness, headache, confusion and purpura. Her blood pressure was 118/72 mmHg. She had a platelet count of 12,000/μL, hemoglobin of 6.8 g/dL, LDH of 4800 U/L, creatinine of 0.9 mg/dL and many fragmented red cells on her peripheral blood smear. Her direct antiglobulin test was negative. She had no evidence for disseminated intravascular coagulation. She recovered with 2 weeks of plasma exchange treatment.

Q What is the most appropriate prognosis for future recurrences of this disorder?

A The disorder will likely not recur
B The disorder will likely recur multiple times
C The disorder will recur with subsequent pregnancy
D The prognosis of recurrence is uncertain

Question 65

A 35-year-old group A male with a body surface area of 2.1 m^2 received a stem cell transplant from his HLA-identical group O brother for second remission AML following a myeloablative preparative regimen. At day 7 his counts are at a nadir, and 1 h after transfusion of a pool of four group A platelet concentrates his platelet count rises from 9000 to 18,000/μL. The following morning his platelet count is 11,000/μL and another transfusion of pooled platelets produces a similar increment. The lymphocytotoxic antibody screen was negative at admission, and he has no splenomegaly.

Q What is the most appropriate action regarding his next platelet transfusion?

A Pooling crossmatch-compatible platelet concentrates
B Pooling only group O platelet concentrates
C Using unmatched apheresis rather than pooled platelet concentrates
D Pooling more than four platelet concentrates
E Using HLA-matched apheresis rather than pooled platelet concentrates

Question 66

A 66-year-old male presents with recurrent hematuria 2 weeks following a transurethral resection of the prostate (TURP). A urinary catheter has been reinserted and shows gross hematuria, and his hemoglobin has dropped by 2 g/dL. Further questioning reveals that he has also bled longer than usual when he cuts himself shaving, and examination shows that he has bruising on his extremities. He denies past bleeding. Laboratory data are as follows:

Prothrombin time	13.3 s (normal 11.2–14.5 s)
APTT	45.9 s (normal 25.4–34.5 s)
Mixing study 1 : 1	35.9 s immediate; 44.8 s at 2 h
Thrombin time	23.3 s (normal 14.8–24.6 s)
Fibrinogen	398 mg/dL
Platelet count	256K/μL

Q What tests will be most helpful in the diagnosis?

A Platelet aggregation studies
B Lupus anticoagulant
C von Willebrand factor assays
D Factor VIII assay
E Factor XII

Question 67

You are asked to see a 69-year-old man with severe coronary artery disease and Rai stage 1 CLL 2 days after three-vessel coronary artery bypass surgery that was complicated by postoperative bleeding at the sternotomy site. He has never been treated for his CLL and was not transfused prior to surgery. The bleeding has stopped but his hemoglobin has decreased to 5.2 g/dL. He has shortness of breath and chest pain. Prior to surgery, the laboratory reported difficulty with blood matching and it now reports that he has positive indirect and direct red cell antibody tests. His postoperative LDH is 351 and his bilirubin is normal. A review of his peripheral blood shows normal platelets and no schistocytes or spherocytes.

Q Which transfusion product would you recommend?

A Washed leukoreduced packed red blood cells
B ABO/Rh-matched 'least-incompatible' packed red blood cells
C Gamma-irradiated packed red blood cells
D Packed red blood cells from an HLA-compatible donor

Question 68

Q Which of the following would promote proliferation of acute myeloid leukemia (AML) blasts?

A Histone deacetylase inhibitor
B All-*trans* retinoic acid
C FLT-3 receptor activator
D Hypomethylating agent

Question 69

A 16-year-old girl is referred for the evaluation of thrombocytopenia. She has a history of learning difficulties. Physical examination reveals short stature (<3rd percentile) without other musculoskeletal abnormalities. Her hemoglobin is 11.4 g/dL, white blood cell count 3.9×10^9/L with absolute neutrophil count 1.9×10^9/L, platelets 18×10^9/L and hemoglobin F percentage 15%. Bone marrow examination reveals hypocellular trilineage myelodysplasia and 8% blasts. Karyotypic analysis reveals trisomy 8 in 4 of 20 metaphases. Peripheral blood mononuclear cells are cultured together with diapoxybutane (DEB). An increased percentage of cells with aberrant chromosomes is noted (DEB positive). The patient has an HLA-identical brother who is hematologically normal and DEB negative.

Q Which of the following is the initial treatment of choice?

A Induction chemotherapy with daunorubicin and cytosine arabinoside (Ara-C)
B Matched sibling allogeneic stem cell transplant with attenuated total body irradiation + cyclophosphamide as conditioning

C Immunosuppression using the combination of antithymocyte globulin and cyclosporine
D Oxymethalone 2 mg/kg/day

Question 70

An 85-year-old woman develops productive cough, high fevers and severe shortness of breath. Physical examination reveals a blood pressure of 80/60 mmHg, heart rate of 120, respiratory rate of 30 and temperature of 38.6°C with diminished breath sounds and crackles over the left lung posteriorly. A chest X-ray shows dense consolidation in the left lung base. Her WBC is 3500/μL with 1300/μL neutrophils and a left-shifted differential, hematocrit 34% and platelet count 63,000/μL. She is admitted to the intensive care unit and antibiotic therapy is begun.

Q Which of the following growth factors would be indicated in this patient?

A Epoetin alfa
B Filgrastim and platelet transfusions
C Filgrastim
D Epoetin alfa plus filgrastim
E No growth factor therapy

Question 71

A 67-year-old Caucasian male is referred for evaluation of hereditary hemochromatosis. He remembers being told 10 years ago that his iron level was elevated. During the past 2 years the patient has developed malaise, arthralgias, new-onset hyperglycemia and right upper quadrant pain. He has no prior history of hepatitis. He drinks 2–3 beers each week and denies consumption of exogenous iron. His only medical problem is moderate high frequency hearing loss. His family history is unknown. A complete blood count is normal. Aspartate aminotransferase (AST) and alanine aminotransferase (ALT) are 330 U/L and 237 U/L, respectively. Iron saturation is 71% and ferritin is 2198 ng/mL. Liver biopsy reveals accumulation of iron primarily in the hepatocytes. Perls stain is 4 + 0. Grade II cirrhosis is also documented.

Q (a) Which of the following genotypic combinations best explains the phenotypic features in this patient with hereditary hemochromatosis?

A H63D/wild-type
B H63D/H63D
C C282Y/wild-type
D C282Y/C282Y
E Wild-type/wild-type

Q (b) Which of the following statements about prognosis and follow-up in this patient is true?

A If he is compliant with phlebotomy, life expectancy will be normal
B Ferritin values should normalize within 6 weeks with weekly phlebotomy
C Malaise may improve as excessive iron is removed
D Life-long screening for hepatoma will not be necessary if phlebotomy is initiated
E Consideration should be given for iron chelation therapy for a more rapid response

Question 72

A 6-year-old boy has been anemic since birth, with hemoglobin ranging from 6 mg/dL to 8 mg/dL. He is microcytic with an MCV of 62 fL. Several male members of his family have had similar hematologic profiles. His marrow reveals ringed sideroblasts when stained with Prussian blue and counterstained with safranin.

Q Which of the following findings would be most likely in this patient?

A Elevated mitochondrial ferritin level
B Low serum ferritin levels
C Reduced free erythrocyte protoporphyrin level
D Normal serum iron level
E Decreased soluble transferrin receptor level

Question 73

A 16-year-old boy with sickle cell anemia (Hb SS) is admitted to the inpatient medical service with what he describes as a typical pain crisis involving his back, arms and legs. He denies any fevers, chills or urinary symptoms. The patient has experienced left-sided chest pain with deep inspiration for the past 24 h. On physical examination, he appears well. Temperature is 37.3°C, blood pressure 123/65 mmHg, heart rate 76 and room air O_2 sat is 96%. He is euvolemic and drinking adequate fluids. Pulmonary examination is unremarkable except for splinting on deep inspiration. Current laboratory data and evaluation include the following:

WBC count	11,400/μL	Urinalysis negative for nitrate and leukocyte esterase
HCT	24%	Chest X-ray: no infiltrates, bibasilar atelectasis
Hb	8.2 g/dL	
Platelet count	234,000/μL	
Reticulocyte count	7%	
Serum electrolytes	Normal	

Q Which of the following is an appropriate next step in the management of this patient?

A Intravenous administration of 0.9% normal saline (NS) at 200 mL/h
B Parenteral administration of meperidine scheduled regularly every 4 h and as needed for pain
C Aggressive incentive spirometry
D Transfusion of 2 units of phenotypically matched red blood cells
E Broad-spectrum antibiotics

Question 74

A 55-year-old man was referred for evaluation of mild anemia and leukopenia. He has a 2-year history of intermittent headaches, diarrhea attributed to irritable bowel syndrome, and chronic dyspepsia attributed to gastroesophageal reflux disease. Current medications include antacids, acetaminophen, ranitidine and dicyclomine. Skin examination is notable for dermatographism and scattered pigmented macules on the chest and abdomen. There are no palpable lymph nodes or hepatosplenomegaly. The hemoglobin is 11.8 g/dL, MCV is 82 fL, reticulocyte count is 80,000/μL, WBC count is 3800/μL, neutrophil count is 1500/μL and the platelet count is 200,000/μL. Marrow aspirate shows normal trilineage hematopoiesis with increased eosinophils and <5% lymphocytes, plasma cells, mast cells and macrophages. Marrow biopsy is normocellular with frequent eosinophils and multifocal paratrabecular aggregates of spindle-shaped cells next to areas of osteosclerosis (see Figure).

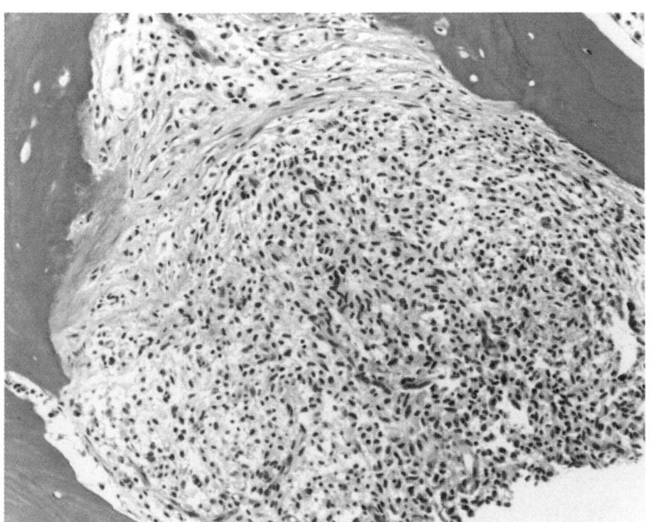

Q Further immunohistologic analysis of the marrow biopsy will most likely identify which of the following?

A Acid-fast + bacilli within marrow histiocytes
B Tartrate-resistant acid phosphatase (TRAP) + hairy cells
C CD30$^+$ Reed–Sternberg cells
D Tryptase + mast cells
E CD20$^+$ large B-cell lymphoma cells

Question 75

A 42-year-old woman with essential thrombocythemia has been treated for the last 3 years with anagrelide and aspirin since having a transient ischemic attack when her platelet count was 1,100,000/μL. Her platelet count has been maintained below 450,000/μL and she has not suffered recurrent thromboembolic events. She missed her menstrual period 2 weeks ago and is confirmed to be pregnant. Past medical history is notable for one uneventful pregnancy and delivery 15 years ago, but two subsequent early trimester miscarriages, both occurring before treatment with anagrelide. She also has major depression with prior hospitalizations, and is currently stable on paroxetine. She and her husband greatly desire another child.

Q What is the most appropriate treatment for this patient through pregnancy and postpartum?

A Aspirin and interferon-α
B Aspirin and plateletpheresis
C Low-molecular-weight heparin and interferon-α
D Low-molecular-weight heparin and plateletpheresis
E Aspirin and anagrelide

Question 76

A 69-year-old man presents to your office with newly diagnosed MDS. Based upon the International Prognostic Scoring System (IPSS), he falls into the intermediate risk-1 prognostic category. He is mildly thrombocytopenic at 90,000/μL and has a symptomatic anemia of 7.7 g/dL. He recently received 2 units of packed red cells. He is in reasonable health but does have a history of type 2 diabetes mellitus and mild renal insufficiency secondary to his diabetes.

Q Which of the following treatments is most appropriate?

A Supportive care with red cell and platelet transfusions
B Treatment with thalidomide

C Combined therapy with erythropoietin/filgrastim in an effort to improve his hemoglobin
D Proceed directly with AML induction chemotherapy in an attempt to induce a complete remission of his disease

Question 77

A 72-year-old man presents with progressive dyspnea on exertion and lightheadedness. He is found to have a hemoglobin of 6.2 g/dL. His white blood cell count is 2500/μL, with an absolute neutrophil count <500/μL. His platelet count is 25,000/μL. A diagnosis of erythroleukemia (FAB M6) is established by bone marrow aspirate and biopsy.

Q Which of the following is the most appropriate induction chemotherapy for this patient?

A Daunorubicin 60 mg/m^2/day for 3 days, plus cytarabine 100 mg/m^2/day for 7 days by continuous infusion
B Daunorubicin 30 mg/m^2/day for 3 days, plus cytarabine 3 g/m^2 twice daily, on days 1–6
C Daunorubicin 30 mg/m^2/day for 3 days, plus cytarabine 500 mg/m^2/day by continuous infusion for 7 days
D Mitoxantrone 10 mg/m^2/day for 5 days, plus etoposide 100 mg/m^2/day for 5 days, plus cytarabine 1 g/m^2/day for 5 days
E Daunorubicin 30 mg/m^2/day for 3 days, plus cytarabine 100 mg/m^2/day for 7 days by continuous infusion, plus gemtuzumab ozogamicin 6 mg/m^2 on day 4

Question 78

A 12-year-old boy presents with abdominal pain. Physical examination shows generalized adenopathy. There is fullness in the right lower quadrant. His liver and spleen are not palpable. Laboratory data include hemoglobin 7.5 g/dL, WBC 9000/μL (5% vacuolated blasts) and platelets 20,000/μL. An abdominal CT shows multiple nodal masses. The bone marrow is replaced by vacuolated blasts with dark blue cytoplasm. Blast surface markers show monoclonal IgM kappa and the karyotype is 46XY, t(8;14).

Q Which of the following is the most appropriate therapy for this patient?

A 3–8 months' systemic chemotherapy
B 3–8 months' systemic chemotherapy plus intrathecal CNS prophylaxis
C 2–3 years' systemic chemotherapy
D 2–3 years' systemic chemotherapy plus intrathecal CNS prophylaxis
E Bone marrow transplant in first complete remission using the best available donor

Question 79

A 42-year-old man with diabetes, hypertension and end-stage renal disease undergoes cadaveric renal transplantation. He is maintained on immunosuppression with tacrolimus, mycophenolate mofetil and prednisone, but 10 months later develops abdominal pain and fever. CT scan reveals a 7-cm left retroperitoneal mass; biopsy is positive for diffuse large B-cell lymphoma. Immunophenotypic markers show monoclonality for lambda light chains, and coexpression of CD10, CD19 and CD20. Reduction of his immunosuppressive regimen leads to no regression in the mass.

Q Which of the following is appropriate therapy for this patient?

A Surgical removal of the graft and discontinuation of immunosuppression
B Combination chemotherapy
C Combination chemotherapy followed by autologous stem cell transplantation
D Rituximab
E Epstein–Barr virus (EBV) antiviral therapy

Question 80

A 37-year-old man with CML in blast crisis received a peripheral blood stem cell transplant from his HLA-identical brother using a busulfan/cyclophosphamide preparative regimen and cyclosporine/methotrexate for graft-versus-host disease (GVHD) prophylaxis. Two days after the stem cells had been infused, the patient complained of right upper quadrant pain. Physical examination showed new tender hepatomegaly, a new fluid wave and peripheral edema. The patient's weight increased 6 kg over a 48-h period. Laboratory findings were significant for both the bilirubin and creatinine tripling over baseline during a 36-h period. A sonogram obtained the following day showed the enlarged liver, ascites and reversal of flow in the portal vein.

Q The most likely diagnosis of the liver dysfunction is:

A Viral hepatitis
B Acute GVHD

C Acute fatty liver
D Veno-occlusive disease (VOD)
E Hematopoiesis occurring in the liver

Question 81

A 19-year-old previously healthy African-American woman had an uncomplicated first pregnancy with delivery of a healthy infant. The following morning she has a severe headache and her vision is blurred. Her blood pressure, which had been normal, is 167/110 mmHg. Her visual acuity is diminished but she has no diplopia or visual field defects. The remainder of her physical examination is normal. Laboratory data are described below:

	Immediately prior to delivery	1 day after delivery
Hemoglobin	12.1 g/dL	11.4 g/dL
Platelet count	249,000/μL	32,000/μL
LDH	127 U/L	642 U/L
Serum creatinine	0.6 mg/dL	0.7 mg/dL
Serum aspartate aminotransferase	37 U/L	427 U/L
Serum alanine aminotransferase	18 U/L	386 U/L

Examination of the blood smear confirms the thrombocytopenia and demonstrates frequent fragmented red cells.

Q Which of the following is the most appropriate management of this patient's condition?

A Observation
B Plasma exchange
C Antibiotics
D Corticosteroids

Question 82

A 55-year-old previously healthy female had increasing fatigue and exercise intolerance for 4 days following gastroenteritis. Her temperature is 38°C, blood pressure 130/75 mmHg and pulse 97. Physical examination is unremarkable aside from pallor, confusion and disorientation for 2 days, and she had a seizure upon admission. Her WBC is 8300/μL, hemoglobin 8.8 g/dL, hematocrit 27%, platelet count 45,000/μL. The reticulocyte count is elevated (absolute count 132,000/μL) with a haptoglobin of <6 and LDH of 875. The direct Coombs test is negative. The peripheral smear shows polychromasia and schistocytes. The PT, APTT, urinalysis, serum electrolytes, creatinine and BUN are normal.

Q What is the optimal initial therapy for this patient?

A Plasma exchange
B Fresh frozen plasma (FFP) transfusion
C Platelet transfusion
D Steroids
E Intravenous immunoglobulin

Question 83

A 34-year-old woman is seen for evaluation of a bleeding disorder before a planned hysterectomy because of severe menorrhagia; she has a past history of postpartum hemorrhage and bleeding after surgical procedures. Her mother also has had bleeding after surgery, but four siblings have no history of bleeding. Her 14-year-old son has no bleeding problems. Physical examination revealed two 7-cm ecchymoses on her lower extremities. Laboratory data are as follows:

Prothrombin time	12.6 s (normal 11.2–14.5 s)
APTT	46.5 s (normal 25.4–34.5 s)
Thrombin time	19.4 s (normal 14.8–24.6 s)
Fibrinogen	356 mg/dL
Platelet count	165,000/μL
Factor VIII activity	8% (50–150%)
VWF antigen	52% (41–132%)
VWF activity (Risto cofactor)	48% (48–144%)
Bleeding time	Normal

Q Which of the following tests would most likely make the diagnosis in this patient?

A A VWF multimer study
B A ristocetin-induced platelet aggregation (RIPA) study
C A binding assay measuring the patient's von Willebrand factor (VWF) binding ability for normal factor VIII
D Platelet aggregation studies
E Lupus anticoagulant assay

Question 84

You are called to the recovery room for a 63-year-old man who has just undergone a four-vessel coronary artery bypass grafting (CABG) procedure. He had a normal preoperative evaluation including a negative bleeding history and family history. Preoperative INR, PTT and platelet count were normal. He was on the bypass oxygenator pump for 75 min and his intraoperative blood loss was 200 mL. Over the last 30 min, 500 mL of bloody fluid drained from a right chest tube and 100 mL of serosanguinous fluid drained from the left chest tube. Examination shows no bleeding in the skin or mucous membranes, at two intravenous sites, a central venous catheter site or his saphenous vein harvest sites. Postoperative laboratory data include a platelet count of 89,000/μL (preoperative count 213,000/μL), INR 1.1 and an APTT of 30 s.

Q Which of the following is the most appropriate response to this patient's postoperative bleeding?

A Return to the operating room for surgical exploration
B Infusion of recombinant factor VIIa and fibrin glue into the chest tube
C Transfusion of two units of single donor apheresis platelets
D Infusion of DDAVP and ε-aminocaproic acid

Question 85

Q Which of the following statements about DNA microarray studies in patients with leukemia is true?

A DNA microarray studies are used to monitor minimal residual disease
B DNA microarray studies require RNA from the malignant cells
C DNA microarray studies are used to diagnose leukemia-associated translocations
D DNA microarray studies assess global patterns of protein levels in leukemia cells

Question 86

A 63-year-old female with a long history of vascular disease and diabetes underwent composite bypass graft surgery of the right external iliac artery. After surgery she was started on clopidogrel. Other medications that she had been taking for at least 15 months were aspirin, lisinopril, furosemide, metoprolol and insulin. At the time of discharge, her blood counts were normal. Six weeks after the surgery, she is admitted with fatigue, shortness of breath on exertion, extensive bruising and mucosal bleeding.

On examination, pallor, bruises and petechiae are noted. There is no splenomegaly or lymphadenopathy. The hemoglobin is 8.2 g/dL, absolute reticulocyte count 25×10^9/L, white cell count 2.9×10^9/L, absolute neutrophil count 0.02×10^9/L and platelet count 3×10^9/L. Liver function tests are normal. Examination of a peripheral blood smear reveals normocytic red blood cells, neutropenia and thrombocytopenia with small platelets. A bone marrow biopsy shows a markedly hypocellular marrow without dysplasia or abnormal cell collections. Transfusion support is started.

Q What is the most appropriate management of the patient at this time?

A Discontinue all medications, give antithymocyte globulin (ATG) and cyclosporine if there is no improvement in her blood counts after 14–21 days
B Discontinue all medications, give ATG and cyclosporine immediately
C Discontinue aspirin and clopidogrel, give ATG and cyclosporine if there is no improvement in her blood counts after 14–21 days
D Discontinue aspirin and clopidogrel, give ATG and cyclosporine immediately
E Discontinue aspirin and clopidogrel, do not treat with immunosuppression

Question 87

A 25-year-old man with recently diagnosed refractory anemia and excess blasts has been hospitalized frequently over the past 2 months for recurrent fever and neutropenia. A decision is made to begin outpatient filgrastim and epoetin alfa in an attempt to improve his peripheral blood counts while searching for an allogeneic stem cell donor. After 5 days of treatment he notes persistent nausea and abdominal pain. On the seventh day of treatment, his abdominal pain increases dramatically. His vital signs include a BP of 90/40 mmHg, heart rate of 140, temperature 37.6°C. Abdominal rigidity, rebound tenderness and diminished bowel sounds are noted. His hematocrit has decreased from 35% to 21% over 2 days. His neutrophil count remains at 200/μL with a total WBC of 2100/μL and a platelet count of 50,000/μL. Lactic dehydrogenase (LDH) and bilirubin are normal. His stools are hemoccult negative and his smear shows hypolobulated neutrophils but is otherwise normal. A direct Coombs test is normal.

Q The most likely diagnosis is:

A Typhlitis
B Splenic rupture
C Appendicitis
D Filgrastim-related fever and muscular pain
E Serum sickness

Question 88

An asymptomatic 42-year-old male sees his primary care physician and requests that he perform iron studies and genetic testing for hereditary hemochromatosis because his father died of cirrhosis at age 67. The patient has two drinks of alcohol socially each week and has no risk factors for hepatitis C. His father drank alcohol excessively. The patient takes a multivitamin daily, but no other exogenous iron. After a lengthy discussion with the patient, the primary care physician complied with his request for hemochromatosis biochemical and genetic screening.

The patient is sent to you for interpretation of the following laboratory data:

Serum iron	95 μg/dL (normal, 42–135 μg/dL)
Serum total iron-binding capacity	303 μg/dL (normal, 225–430 μg/dL)
Transferrin saturation	31% (normal, 20–50%)
Ferritin	267 ng/mL (normal, 30–400 ng/mL)

Genetic results read as follows:

No copies of the C282Y mutation are detected upon examination of the *HFE* locus on chromosome 6
A single copy of the H63D mutation is noted upon examination of the *HFE* locus on chromosome 6

Q Which of the following statements is true (assuming he continues with his current lifestyle)?

A He will most likely develop clinical iron overload later in life
B He has a 25% chance of passing on the H63D mutation to his children
C An aggressive phlebotomy program aiming to decrease serum ferritin values to below 50 ng/mL should be initiated
D The chance of developing clinical iron overload is less than 5%
E Given the rarity of this mutation, no accurate predictions can be made concerning future risk of iron overload

Question 89

A 12-year-old Israeli girl has had a macrocytic anemia for her entire life, with hemoglobin levels in the 8–9 mg/dL range. She is also noted to have gallstones and a serum ferritin of 733 ng/mL. Her marrow reveals erythroid dysplasia characterized by multinuclear erythroid precursors with occasional pairs of nuclei connected by thin chromatin bridges. In some cells, there is cytoplasm separating the nuclear chromatin fragments giving the nucleus a spongy appearance.

Q An abnormality of which of the following erythrocyte components is responsible for this disorder?

A Spectrin
B Ankyrin
C Nuclear membrane
D Membrane glycoproteins
E Na^+/K^+ ATPase

Question 90

An 18-year-old woman with sickle cell anemia (Hb SS) comes to you for a second opinion before starting hydroxyurea therapy. Her recent medical history is significant for 4–5 yearly admissions for uncomplicated pain crisis and a single episode of acute chest syndrome 2 years ago. She suffered a stroke at age 4 but has no residual abnormalities. She has received multiple previous blood transfusions and has known alloantibodies to blood groups C, e and Kell. She is not on a chronic transfusion program.

Q During your consultation, you inform the patient:

A Hydroxyurea has teratogenic potential and contraception is required
B Hydroxyurea has been shown to reduce hospital admissions but not acute chest syndrome
C The risk of leukemia does not need to be discussed as hydroxyurea has never been implicated as a cause of leukemia
D Hydroxyurea is only indicated for patients older than 21 years of age
E She has no current clinical indication for initiation of hydroxyurea therapy

Question 91

A 5-week-old male presents with 1 day of fever and cellulitis around the umbilicus. The baby appears ill with fever and grunting respirations. The umbilical cord stump is present with induration and erythema around the site. The hemoglobin is 11.8 g/dL, MCV is 94 fL, platelet count is 210,000/μL and the WBC count is 2300/μL, with 77% lymphocytes, 20% monocytes, 1% neutrophils and 2% band forms. The infant is admitted and treated with broad-spectrum intravenous antibiotics. He becomes afebrile by the second hospital day. After a follow-up CBC shows no significant changes, a bone marrow aspirate is performed, which reveals trilineage hematopoiesis with a maturation arrest at the myelocyte–metamyelocyte stage. A presumptive diagnosis of severe congenital neutropenia (SCN) is made and recombinant G-CSF (filgrastim) is prescribed at a dosage of 5 μg/kg/day.

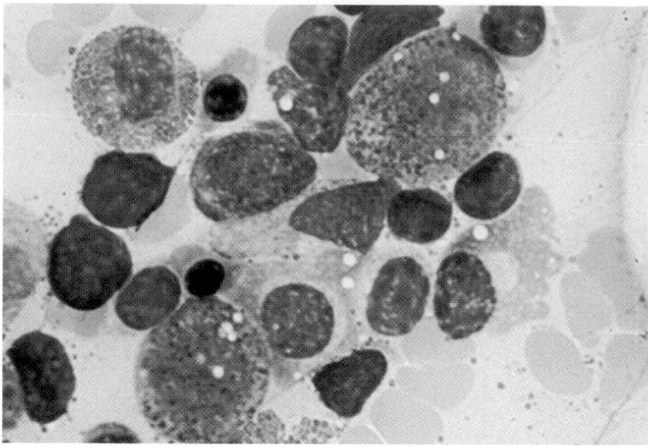

Q Which of the following statements about this child's response to this therapy and his long-term management is true?

A The patient will respond to therapy with a prompt rise in the neutrophil count and this therapy should be continued long term

B The patient will likely respond to therapy and it should be discontinued when the acute infection has resolved

C The patient will have an unpredictable response to therapy, dose adjustment may be necessary, and therapy should be continued long term

D The patient is likely to respond in the short term, but stem cell transplantation from an HLA-matched unrelated donor is the preferred long-term management

Question 92

A 62-year-old man with a 5-year history of untreated essential thrombocythemia (ET) complains of recurrent epistaxis and easy bruising. He denies visual complaints, constitutional symptoms, abdominal fullness or early satiety. His disease course to date has been unremarkable, with a platelet count in the range of 800,000–950,000/μL. He has never suffered a thromboembolic event. He takes multivitamins and acetaminophen, but avoids aspirin and nonsteroidal anti-inflammatory agents because they induce bruising. Physical examination reveals ecchymoses on the distal extremities and dried blood in the left nares. The spleen is palpable 2 cm below the left costal margin. Laboratory data are as follows:

Hematocrit	38%
MCV	95 fL
Leukocyte count	9800/μL
Platelet count	1,650,000/μL
Prothrombin time/INR	12 s/1.1
Activated partial thromboplastin time (APTT)	65 s (2.2 times control)
PTT after 1 : 1 mix	32 s (1.1 times control)
Thrombin time (TT)	22 s (normal)

Q Which of the following is the most likely cause of this patient's bleeding complications?

A Qualitative platelet dysfunction

B Acquired factor VIII inhibitor

C Acquired von Willebrand disease

D Lupus anticoagulant

Question 93

Q Which of the following statements about 5-azacitidine therapy in intermediate-2 or high-risk MDS is true?

A It induces a complete remission in most treated patients

B It is likely to result in a complete cytogenetic response

C It improves survival and delays progression to AML compared with supportive care alone

D It results in a 50% 10-year disease-free survival rate

Question 94

A 41-year-old woman seeks medical attention because of persistent low-grade fever, cough, mild hemoptysis and spontaneous lower extremity bruising. Laboratory studies show a white blood cell count of 45,000/μL with 60% primitive mononuclear cells in the peripheral blood. The serum fibrinogen is 90 mg/dL. A bone marrow aspirate and biopsy reveal acute myeloid leukemia with abnormal-appearing eosinophils.

Q Which of the following statements regarding this patient is true?

A Molecular studies are likely to show a fusion of the *PML* and *RARα* genes

B Induction chemotherapy with daunorubicin 60 mg/m^2/day for 3 days plus all-*trans* retinoic acid (ATRA) is likely to induce a remission

C Molecular studies are likely to show a fusion of the *MYH11* and *CBFβ* genes
D Cytogenetic studies are likely to demonstrate the t(8;21) translocation
E Cytogenetic studies are likely to demonstrate the t(15;17) translocation

Question 95

An 18-year-old male presents with increasing fatigue and cough. CBC is normal but a chest X-ray reveals an 8-cm anterior mediastinal mass. CT scans confirm the chest mass but show no other abnormalities. Biopsy of the mass is consistent with precursor T-cell lymphoblastic lymphoma. Bone marrow biopsy reveals 10% blast forms.

Q Which of the following is appropriate therapy for precursor T-cell lymphoblastic lymphoma in an adult?

A CHOP chemotherapy for 6–8 cycles
B ALL-type regimen with intrathecal central nervous system prophylaxis
C CHOP chemotherapy for 6–8 cycles followed by radiation to the mediastinum
D ALL-type regimen with intrathecal chemotherapy only if cerebrospinal fluid cytology is positive
E Immediate high-dose therapy with autologous stem cell transplantation

Question 96

A 74-year-old woman is found to have a 2.5-cm left lower lobe lung nodule on chest X-ray, appearing since her last annual examination 1 year ago. She is a nonsmoker and has no cough, chest pain or other respiratory symptoms. There is no peripheral adenopathy, laboratory studies are normal, and CT scans of the chest and abdomen are negative aside from the lung nodule. The lesion is deemed inaccessible for fine needle aspiration or bronchoscopic biopsy. She undergoes complete wedge resection; pathology is consistent with mucosa-associated lymphoid tissue (MALT) lymphoma.

Q Which of the following is appropriate follow-up for this patient?

A Periodic physical examinations and imaging studies
B PET scan
C Rituximab
D Chemotherapy plus rituximab
E Radiation therapy to ipsilateral hilar and mediastinal nodes

Question 97

A CMV-positive 31-year-old man received a matched unrelated donor transplant for Philadelphia (Ph) chromosome-positive ALL in first complete remission. The patient did well through the initial transplant and was discharged home at 30 days post-transplant with full engraftment on prophylactic antibiotics, tapering steroids and cyclosporine. One week after discharge, the patient develops fever, diarrhea, nausea and vomiting. The patient is brought to clinic with these symptoms and receives intravenous fluids for 3 days until the symptoms subside. The patient reports that he has been unable to take his medications for 3 days. One week later, the patient returns with a rash and diarrhea.

Q All of the following tests are reasonable to evaluate the patient *except*:

A Skin biopsy of the rash
B Stool culture
C Colonoscopy with biopsy
D Cyclosporine level
E Chimerism studies

Question 98

A 72-year-old previously healthy Caucasian woman is admitted to the hospital following several days of increasing confusion, dyspnea and weakness. On examination, her vital signs are normal except for a respiratory rate of 36. Several petechiae are present about her lower legs and ankles. A hard 3-cm mass is felt in her right breast. There are no focal neurologic abnormalities. The remainder of the examination is normal.

Laboratory data demonstrate hemoglobin 8.2 g/dL, white blood cell count 18,200/μL, platelet count 22,000/μL; examination of the blood smear demonstrates 18 nucleated red cells/100 white cells, frequent fragmented and teardrop red cells, and the presence of myelocytes and metamyelocytes. There is no evidence for disseminated intravascular coagulopathy (DIC). Serum LDH 6250 U/L, serum creatinine 2.1 mg/dL.

Chest X-ray and brain CT scan are normal; spiral CT scan of the lungs demonstrates multiple pulmonary emboli. Echocardiogram demonstrates right ventricular dilation.

Bilateral lower extremity ultrasound examinations demonstrate no deep venous thrombosis.

Q Which of the following is the most appropriate management for this patient?

A Plasma exchange and defer the evaluation of the breast mass
B Bone marrow biopsy and schedule a biopsy of the breast mass
C Placement of an inferior vena cava filter; schedule a biopsy of the breast mass
D Therapy with vitamin B_{12} and folic acid and schedule a biopsy of the breast mass
E Transfusion of red cells and platelets and schedule a biopsy of the breast mass

Question 99

A 110-kg male accident victim had a crush injury to his right leg that fractured the femur and lacerated the femoral artery. He received a total of 25 units of packed red blood cells and 11 liters of Ringer lactate during the 5-h surgery. As they began to close the incision, the surgeons noticed diffuse bleeding not easily controlled by cauterization. Laboratory data showed WBC 5200/μL, hemoglobin 8.9 g/dL, hematocrit 28%, platelet count 77,000/μL, PT 23.7 s, INR 1.97 and APTT 61 s.

Q Which blood product would be optimal to help this patient's bleeding?

A Platelet concentrates
B Whole blood
C Fresh frozen plasma
D Cryoprecipitate
E Packed red blood cells

Question 100

A 68-year-old woman presents to her physician with complaints of fatigue and easy bruising. On physical examination she has multiple 1–2-cm cervival and axillary lymph nodes and her spleen is palpated 2 cm below her costal margin. Initial laboratory evaluation reveals a hemoglobin of 9.2 g/dL, WBC of 6500/μL with a normal differential and a platelet count of 186,000/μL. Her reticulocyte count is 42,000/μL and her sedimentation rate is 98 mm/h. A clonal population of B cells is identified by flow cytometry on the bone marrow aspirate specimen. The B cells are CD20, CD38 and IgM kappa positive. They are negative for CD5, CD10 and CD23.

Q The most likely diagnosis is:

A Chronic lymphocytic leukemia
B Multiple myeloma
C Mantle cell lymphoma
D Lymphoplasmacytic lymphoma

Question 101

Q Which of the following is true concerning restriction fragment length polymorphisms (RFLPs)?

A RFLPs directly detect pathogenic point mutations in most diagnostic applications
B RFLP analysis is an application of the Western blot technique
C RFLPs are often located in intronic or intergenic sequences
D RFLPs detect acquired somatic mutations in individuals

Question 102

A 70-year-old male presents with moderately severe epistaxis. He is being treated with lisinopril for hypertension. On examination, he is noted to have petechiae on the extremities and in the oropharynx. He does not have a palpable spleen or lymphadenopathy. The hemoglobin is 7.2 g/dL, absolute reticulocyte count 20×10^9/L, white cell count 2.9×10^9/L, absolute neutrophil count 1.0×10^9/L and platelet count 80×10^9/L. The peripheral blood smear shows macrocytic red blood cells, hypogranular neutrophils and a few giant platelets.

Q The most likely cause of the epistaxis is:

A Lisinopril-induced platelet dysfunction
B Thrombocytopenia
C Hypertension
D Platelet dysfunction associated with myelodysplastic syndrome
E Platelet dysfunction associated with aplastic anemia

Question 103

A 50-year-old man develops extensive small cell lung cancer. His oncologist considers treatment with either cytoxan, Adriamycin and etoposide (CAE) or etoposide plus cisplatin. Both of the regimens produce comparable response rates and overall survival and are generally equivalent in toxicity profile, but CAE produces a 40% chance of fever without cytokine support while the etoposide plus cisplatin regimen produces a much lower rate of febrile neutropenia.

Q Which of the following approaches is preferred?

A CAE plus filgrastim for the first cycle; dose reduce for the second cycle if febrile neutropenia occurs with the first cycle
B Etoposide plus cisplatin for the first cycle; add filgrastim if febrile neutropenia occurs with the first cycle
C Etoposide plus cisplatin for the first cycle; if febrile neutropenia occurs, dose reduce for the second cycle
D CAE for the first cycle; if febrile neutropenia occurs, add filgrastim until neutropenia resolves; dose reduce for the second cycle

Question 104

A 27-year-old female is transferred from a referring hospital for further evaluation of crampy abdominal pain. The patient has required several hospital admissions for similar episodes of abdominal pain since she began menstruating at age 12 years. Extensive gastrointestinal evaluation, including laboratory, endoscopic and imaging studies, has repeatedly been nondiagnostic. She currently complains of crampy mid-abdominal pain, nausea and vomiting. She has no history of skin lesions. Her friends describe her as emotionally labile. Medications include oral contraception and a daily multivitamin. Physical examination is significant only for a tender abdomen, but no rebound or guarding is appreciated. Electrolytes including hepatic enzymes, amylase and lipase levels all return normal. Computed tomography (CT) of the abdomen is unremarkable, except for a nonspecific bowel gas pattern.

Q Which of the following studies should be carried out next in this patient?

A Urine uroporphyrin levels
B Random skin biopsy
C Red cell porphobilinogen (PBG) deaminase levels
D Urine δ-aminolevulinic acid (ALA) and PBG levels
E Push enteroscopy

Question 105

A 55-year-old woman with no previous medical problems and on no medications presents with increasing fatigue and weakness of several months' duration. Her review of systems is positive for a weight gain of 40 lbs over the previous 2 years. A complete blood count (CBC) shows a hemoglobin of 7 g/dL and an MCV of 108 fL. Serum vitamin B_{12} level is 100 ng/L and the red blood cell (RBC) folate is within the normal range. A bone marrow examination shows changes consistent with megaloblastic anemia. Iron stores are normal. She is diagnosed with vitamin B_{12} deficiency and begun on vitamin B_{12} 1000 μg/day intramuscularly for 1 week and then weekly for 1 month. She returns for follow-up CBC after 1 month of treatment. On her return visit, her hemoglobin is 8 g/dL, and a corrected reticulocyte count is 2.0%.

Q What laboratory study is most likely to reveal the cause of the patient's persistent anemia?

A Measurement of serum ferritin
B Measurement of serum lactate dehydrogenase (LDH)
C Direct antiglobulin test
D Measurement of serum thyroid-stimulating hormone
E Measurement of serum aminotransferases

Question 106

A 55-year-old woman with a history of rheumatoid arthritis complains of a 2-week history of fatigue and yellowing of her skin and eyes. She is afebrile and normotensive. On physical examination, she has deformities of the metacarpophalangeal joints and obvious scleral icterus. The spleen is palpated 3 cm below the costal margin. No adenopathy or hepatomegaly is appreciated. Laboratory data and peripheral blood smear (see Figure) are shown below:

WBC count	6800/μL
Hematocrit	26%
Hemoglobin	8.3 g/dL
Platelet count	167,000/μL
Reticulocyte count (uncorrected)	14%
Bilirubin, total	5.4 mg/dL
Bilirubin, direct	0.8 mg/dL
LDH	1500 U/L

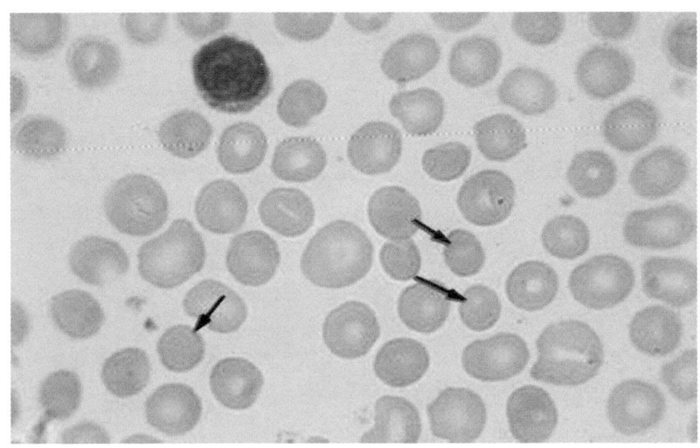

Q Which one of the following results would be expected on further laboratory and blood bank testing?

A Strongly positive cold agglutinin titer
B Normal osmotic fragility test
C Direct antiglobulin test (DAT) positive for C3, but not IgG
D Difficulty in initial attempts at performing an accurate type and screen

Question 107

A 2-year-old girl presents for evaluation of chronic drainage from her right ear that has persisted for 3 months despite multiple courses of oral antibiotics. The past medical history includes 1–2 episodes of uncomplicated otitis media during the first 18 months of life. The physical examination reveals a slender child in no distress with a purulent discharge in the right ear canal. She also has a crusted rash on her trunk and bilateral anterior cervical and axillary adenopathy, with the largest lymph node measuring 2 × 2 cm. The left ear and remainder of the physical examination are normal. The CBC shows a WBC count of 8000/μL with a normal differential, hemoglobin 11.6 g/dL and a platelet count of 381,000/μL. An X-ray of the skull reveals a lytic lesion in the left mastoid bone.

Q Which of the following is the most appropriate next step in the management of this patient?

A Full body soft tissue and bone imaging studies
B Biopsy of an enlarged left cervical lymph node
C Curettage of the involved mastoid bone
D Radiation therapy of the involved mastoid bone
E Multi-agent chemotherapy

Question 108

A 59-year-old man is referred for evaluation of anemia, low-grade fever and weight loss. He has a history of hypertension and hypercholesterolemia. He takes lovastatin and lisinopril. He denies respiratory symptoms, abdominal pain, melena and hematochezia. Physical examination is notable for a weight of 95 kg and mild pallor. The spleen tip is palpable 2 cm below the left costal margin and there is no obvious hepatomegaly. Small (≤1 cm) lymph nodes are felt in the inguinal regions. Stool is guaiac negative. Laboratory data are as follows:

Hematocrit	33%
MCV	88 fL
Leukocyte count	8800/μL
Platelet count	140,000/μL
Absolute reticulocyte count	100,000/μL
Peripheral blood smear	Occasional nucleated and teardrop erythrocytes, neutrophilic bands and giant platelets
Ferritin	180 μg/dL
Uric acid	10.0 mg/dL
Lactate dehydrogenase	390 U/L
Vitamin B_{12} and folate	Both normal
Direct antiglobulin test	Negative
Antinuclear antibody	Positive at 1 : 40

Marrow biopsy shows hypercellularity with myeloid and megakaryocytic hyperplasia and grade 2+ reticulin fibrosis.

Q All of the following are potential diagnoses in this patient *except*:

A Idiopathic myelofibrosis (agnogenic myeloid metaplasia)
B Non-Hodgkin lymphoma
C Myelodysplastic syndrome
D Primary autoimmune myelofibrosis
E Metastatic carcinoma

Question 109

A 38-year-old male presents with trilineage cytopenias, but no myeloblasts in the peripheral blood. He has recently required transfusions because of the symptomatic cytopenias. On bone marrow examination, he is found to have a hypercellular marrow with 15% myeloid blasts. He is also found to have a complex karyotype. He has three siblings, one of whom is HLA-identical.

Q Which of the following would be the most appropriate therapy to recommend for this patient?

A Allogeneic stem cell transplant using an HLA-identical donor
B Supportive care with transfusions and antibiotic prophylaxis
C Immunosuppressive therapy with antithymocyte globulin (ATG) and cyclosporine
D Autologous stem cell transplant

Question 110

A 75-year-old man is brought to the emergency room by his family where he complains of headache and visual change. A careful history reveals progressive dyspnea on exertion, generalized fatigue and spontaneous bruising. His laboratory studies show a white blood cell count of 480,000/μL, of which 80% are reported to be blasts. His hemoglobin is 7.2 g/dL and his platelet count is 18,000/μL. A CT scan of the head shows a small intracerebral hemorrhage.

Q Which of the following is the most appropriate next step in the management of this patient?

A Chemotherapy with daunorubicin and cytarabine
B Emergent leukapheresis followed the next day by chemotherapy with daunorubicin and cytarabine
C Emergent leukapheresis plus hydroxyurea
D Emergent cranial irradiation, plus hydroxyurea, followed the next day by chemotherapy with daunorubicin and cytarabine
E Emergent cranial irradiation, plus emergent leukapheresis and hydroxyurea, followed the next day by chemotherapy with daunorubicin and cytarabine

Question 111

A 24-year-old woman is referred for evaluation of fatigue and bruising. She is pale and has petechiae on her extremities. WBC is 80,000/μL, hemoglobin 7.2 g/dL and platelets 12,000/μL. Bone marrow biopsy is hypercellular with a predominance of blasts; flow cytometry confirms precursor-B ALL. Cytogenetics reveals a t(12;21) translocation.

Q Which of the following is a favorable prognostic factor in a young adult with ALL?

A Pre-B-cell phenotype
B High white blood cell count
C Slow initial response to prednisone
D Thrombocytopenia
E t(12;21)

Question 112

A 32-year-old man is referred for evaluation of a left neck mass. He first noted a small 'knot' in the left neck about 3 weeks ago, but states it has rapidly increased since that time. Examination confirms a nontender, 4 × 6-cm, left supraclavicular mass but no other peripheral adenopathy. CBC, chemistries and LDH are normal. Biopsy of the mass shows a diffuse, small, noncleaved cell lymphoma with a high mitotic rate, a 'starry sky' pattern and a $CD10^+$, B-cell phenotype. CT scans show no pathologic adenopathy aside from the left supraclavicular mass. Bone marrow biopsy is negative.

Q Which of the following therapies is indicated?

A Combination chemotherapy plus central nervous system (CNS) chemoprophylaxis
B Combination chemotherapy plus CNS chemoprophylaxis if cerebrospinal fluid is positive for lymphoma
C Autologous stem cell transplantation in first remission
D Allogeneic stem cell transplantation in first remission

Question 113

A 2-year-old girl presents to her local pediatrician. She is somewhat irritable and her mother notes that she is becoming paler. On physical examination she has a palpable mass and by CT scan is noted to have a calcified mass arising from the region of her right kidney. The surgeon is unable to resect the tumor but is able to provide you with a biopsy that reveals a small round blue cell tumor. Bone marrow biopsy reveals a similar appearing cell.

Q In addition to intensive chemotherapy, which of the following is the most appropriate management of this patient?

A Intensive chemotherapy, radiation therapy and/or surgery and differentiation therapy
B Intensive chemotherapy, allogeneic transplant and differentiation therapy
C Intensive chemotherapy, autologous transplant and differentiation therapy
D Intensive chemotherapy, radiation therapy and/or surgery, autologous transplant and differentiation therapy

Question 114

Q Which of the following viruses has the highest risk of transmission through blood transfusion?

A HTLV-1/2
B HCV

C HIV
D HBV

Question 115

A 47-year-old nurse is referred for evaluation of splenomegaly. On questioning the patient you note that she has lost 10% of her body weight over a period of 6 months and that she complains of fatigue. On examination you note two cervical nodes measuring 1×2 cm. A CT scan of the chest, abdomen and pelvis confirms splenomegaly and shows mild diffuse retroperitoneal adenopathy. Her bone marrow biopsy is involved with lymphoma. The clonal B lymphocytes are CD20, CD5 and kappa light chain positive. CD23 and CD10 are not expressed.

Q Which of the following statements about this patient's condition is true?

A The clonal B cells are typically BCL-6 positive
B The clonal B cells are typically cyclin D1 positive
C The t(14;18)(q32;q21) is typical of this lymphoma
D The t(2;8)(q11;q24) is typical of this lymphoma

Question 116

You are asked to see a 65-year-old woman for progressive venous thrombosis and an ischemic left foot. Fourteen days ago she underwent debulking surgery for stage IIIA ovarian cancer. Two days after surgery she had acute left leg swelling. A deep venous thrombosis (DVT) was diagnosed by Doppler ultrasonography. She was treated with intravenous unfractionated heparin (UFH) with an adequate rise in her APTT; warfarin was started 7 days ago. Two days ago, the left leg swelling increased and her left foot became cold and blue. A repeat Doppler ultrasound showed extension of the venous thrombosis but no evidence of arterial clot. Arteriography also showed no evidence of arterial thrombosis. The INR was 2.1 and the platelet count was 52,000/μL; prior to instituting heparin the platelet count was 230,000/μL. UFH was discontinued.

Q Which of the following would be the most appropriate next step in the management of this patient?

A Start a low-molecular-weight heparin; increase the warfarin dose
B Increase the warfarin dose only
C Stop warfarin; start a direct thrombin inhibitor
D Stop warfarin; start a thrombolytic agent

Question 117

Q In an RT-PCR assay, amplification of contaminating genomic DNA can be minimized by:

A Including a negative control
B Using primers designed with 50% G-C content
C Using PCR primers that span a large intron
D Treating with RNAse before reverse transcription

Question 118

A 37-year-old male who has had decreased exercise tolerance for 3 months is noted to have pancytopenia. He is not taking any medications. On examination, pallor is noted. He does not have any lymphadenopathy or splenomegaly. The hemoglobin is 5.2 g/dL, absolute reticulocyte count 30×10^9/L, white cell count 1.8×10^9/L, absolute neutrophil count 0.7×10^9/L and platelet count 28×10^9/L. The bone marrow biopsy cellularity is 10% and the bone marrow aspirate smear reveals hypocellular spicules with no evidence of dysplasia or abnormal cells. Bone marrow cytogenetics is normal.

He has three siblings, one of whom is a complete HLA match. One of the siblings is an active blood donor and the patient states that if he is to receive a blood transfusion, he would like to receive blood products from his sibling to decrease the risk of acquiring a transfusion-related infection.

Q Which of the following would be appropriate management of this patient?

A Transfusion support with sibling-derived irradiated leukocyte-depleted blood products to increase the hemoglobin to 8–10 g/dL
B Transfusion support with nonsibling-derived irradiated leukocyte-depleted blood products to increase the hemoglobin to 8–10 g/dL
C Transfusion support with sibling-derived nonirradiated nonleukocyte-depleted blood products
D Erythropoietin and granulocyte colony-stimulating factor injections and avoidance of all blood products

Question 119

Q Which of the following statements about the relative effects of pegfilgrastim and filgrastim as an adjunct to myelosuppressive chemotherapy is true?

A Pegfilgrastim decreases the mortality rate and improves the remission rate more than filgrastim therapy

B Pegfilgrastim reduces the likelihood of hospitalization for neutropenic fever compared with filgrastim
C Pegfilgrastim has fewer side-effects than filgrastim therapy
D One dose of pegfilgrastim provides the same neutrophil support as 11 daily doses of filgrastim

Question 120

A 38-year-old female is known to have acute intermittent porphyria (AIP). She experienced frequent episodes of crampy abdominal pain soon after menarche and throughout her teenage years, but has been well for several years. She is not aware of her prior treatment regimens. She presents to the emergency room this afternoon with crampy non-localizing abdominal pain that she describes as similar to her prior episodes. She has recently been started on oral contraception, but cannot recall the name of the product. On examination, her abdomen is diffusely tender, but there is no rebound or guarding. Laboratory and radiographic studies are unremarkable.

Q The most appropriate initial management of this patient should include:

A Surgical consultation
B Intravenous panhemitin
C Intravenous dextrose and narcotic analgesics
D Psychiatric referral

Question 121

A 60-year-old female presents with fatigue and dyspnea on exertion. Her past medical history is only significant for a deep venous thrombosis (DVT) and pulmonary embolism (PE) that occurred 2 years prior to this presentation. Following 6 months of warfarin therapy, oral anticoagulation was discontinued. One year later she experienced a recurrent DVT for which she remains on warfarin at the time of this presentation. She is not on any other medications and has no other medical history. She has no family history of anemia or thrombosis. She denies any signs of bleeding such as hematemesis or melena.

A CBC shows a hemoglobin of 6.6 g/dL, with an MCV of 96 fL. Her platelet count is 115,000/μL and her absolute neutrophil count is 2200/μL. A peripheral smear shows ovalocytes and a rare hypersegmented neutrophil. Her international normalized ratio (INR) is 2.1.

Q (a) The most likely cause of her anemia is:

A Vitamin B_{12} deficiency
B Paroxysmal nocturnal hemoglobinuria
C Warm antibody hemolytic anemia
D Iron deficiency resulting from blood loss
E Anemia of chronic disease

Q (b) The most likely underlying cause of hypercoagulability in this patient is:

A Antithrombin deficiency
B Paroxysmal nocturnal hemoglobinuria
C Hyperhomocysteinemia
D Venous stasis disease
E Older age

Question 122

A 38-year-old African-American man is admitted 3 weeks after cadaveric renal transplantation complaining of fatigue, dyspnea and dark urine. Physical examination is significant for scleral icterus and lack of lymphadenopathy or hepatosplenomegaly. Prior to transplantation the hematocrit value was maintained at 34% with erythropoietin administration. His post-transplant medications include cyclosporine, prednisone at 20 mg/day, trimethoprim-sulfamethoxazole and acyclovir. He does not smoke tobacco and denies alcohol consumption or other illicit drug use. Laboratory evaluation and peripheral blood smear (see Figure) are shown below.

Hb	5.8 g/dL
Hct	18%
Platelet count	267,000 μL
Reticulocyte count	6%
LDH	1332 IU/L
Coombs test	Negative

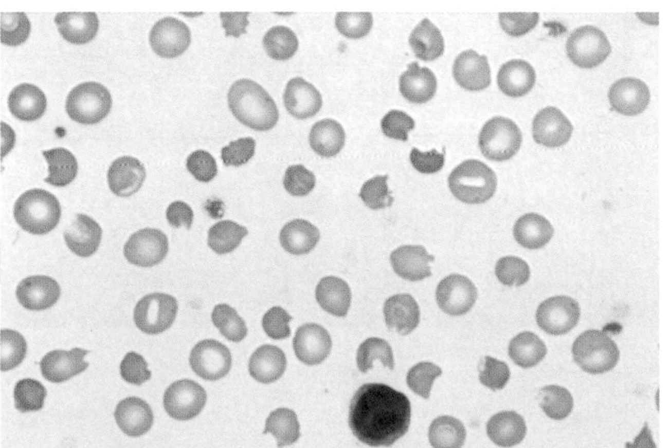

Q The next step in the management of this patient should include:

A Stop cyclosporine
B Begin plasma exchange therapy
C Stop trimethoprim-sulfamethoxazole
D Send a glucose-6-phosphate dehydrogenase (G6PD) assay and await results
E Increase the prednisone dosage to 60 mg/day

Question 123

A 5-year-old boy is admitted for sinusitis. Three days earlier, he was noted to have a fever that was associated with pain over the right cheek. This progressed over 24 h, and he was begun on oral antibiotics after an X-ray revealed opacification of the right maxillary sinus. However, he showed no improvement and was therefore admitted for parenteral antibiotic therapy. The past medical history is remarkable for multiple episodes of otitis media during the first 2 years of life, which ultimately resulted in polyethylene tube placement. He has had two admissions for pneumonia. He also had *Staphylococcus aureus* isolated from a purulent abscess that developed on his thigh at age 3 years, which resolved after a 2-week course of intravenous antibiotics. The physical examination reveals a slender cooperative boy who is febrile but not in acute distress. There is localized tenderness over the right maxilla but little erythema or induration. His ear canals are clear and both tympanic membranes are scarred with myringotomy tubes in place. Shoddy cervical and inguinal adenopathy is detected. His skin is clear and there is a large well-healed scar on the right thigh. The CBC shows a WBC count of 22,000/μL with 88% neutrophils and 5% bands, hemoglobin 9.9 g/dL and a platelet count of 608,000/μL.

Q Which laboratory test is most likely to indicate the underlying hematologic diagnosis?

A A bone marrow aspirate and biopsy
B Nitroblue tetrazolium (NBT) test
C Analysis for a mutation in the *SBDS* gene
D Serum ferritin
E Studies of neutrophil chemotaxis

Question 124

A 49-year-old woman with a 5-year history of idiopathic myelofibrosis (agnogenic myeloid metaplasia) complains of progressive shortness of breath, worsening fatigue and involuntary weight loss. Hydroxyurea has been used for the last 3 years to control splenomegaly and epoetin alfa has been started recently for anemia. She has not had bleeding or thromboembolic complications. Physical examination reveals absent breath sounds and dullness to percussion over the lower two-thirds of the left lung field and splenomegaly extending into the pelvis. The liver edge is 2 cm below the right costal margin. CT scans reveal a large left pleural effusion with pleural-based masses, massive homogeneous splenomegaly and mild hepatomegaly. Therapeutic thoracentesis is carried out and biopsy of the left parietal pleural mass reveals trilineage extramedullary hematopoiesis. The patient's 46-year-old sister is determined to be an HLA-identical match to the patient. Laboratory data are as follows:

Hematocrit	25%
MCV	106 fL
Leukocyte count	11,700/μL
Platelet count	40,000/μL
White cell differential	Neutrophils 5000/μL
	Bands 800/μL
	Immature myeloid precursors 1900/μL
	Blasts 300/μL
	Monocytes 700/μL
	Lymphocytes 2300/μL
	Eosinophils and basophils 700/μL

Marrow evaluation: 'dry tap' aspirate. Biopsy reveals 80% replacement with grade 4+ fibrosis. Cytogenetics reveals a new trisomy 12 clonal abnormality.

Q Which of the following is the most appropriate management strategy for this patient?

A Low-dose thalidomide and proceed with myeloablative stem cell transplantation
B Irradiation of the left hemithorax and proceed with myeloablative stem cell transplantation
C Irradiation of the left hemithorax followed by low-dose thalidomide
D Interferon-α and proceed with myeloablative stem cell transplantation
E Irradiation of the left hemithorax followed by interferon-α

Question 125

A 67-year-old female presents with complaints of left upper quadrant pain and has splenomegaly on examination. Evaluation of the peripheral blood reveals an HCT of 30%, platelet count of 50,000/μL and a WBC count of 45,000/μL, with 60% monocytes. Bone scan reveals trilineage dysmorphology, increased monocytes and 8% myeloblasts. Cytogenetic studies reveal the t(5;12).

Q Which of the following is the most appropriate therapy for this patient?

A AML-type induction chemotherapy
B Allogeneic stem cell transplant
C Imatinib mesylate therapy
D Palliative transfusion support

Question 126

A 42-year-old lawyer comes to medical attention because of fatigue and spontaneous bruising. His white blood cell count is found to be 48,000/μL, hemoglobin 8.3 g/dL and platelet count 18,000/μL. A bone marrow aspirate and biopsy reveal acute promyelocytic leukemia. Cytogenetic analysis shows the t(15;17) translocation. Molecular analysis demonstrates the presence of PML-RARα fusion protein. The patient is given a combination of all-*trans* retinoic acid (ATRA) daily, 45 mg/m^2/day in divided doses, followed 3 days later by daunorubicin 60 mg/m^2/day for 3 days. On day 5 of treatment, the patient complains of marked shortness of breath and a chest radiograph reveals bilateral fluffy infiltrates and small bilateral pleural effusions.

Q Which of the following is the most appropriate immediate management of this patient?

A Start cytarabine
B Discontinue ATRA
C Discontinue ATRA and start cytarabine
D Start dexamethasone and cytarabine
E Discontinue ATRA and start dexamethasone

Question 127

A 64-year-old woman presents with headache, blurry vision and bruising. The physical examination reveals petechiae and retinal hemorrhage with WBC 110,000/μL, Hb 7.8 g/dL, and platelets 8000/μL. The peripheral blood smear shows a predominance of small blasts, and flow cytometry is consistent with pre-B-cell ALL.

Q All of the following are indicated in this patient *except*:

A Aggressive fluid hydration and tumor lysis prophylaxis
B 3–4 cycles of consolidation therapy with high-dose cytarabine
C Intensive multi-agent combination chemotherapy
D Intrathecal CNS prophylaxis
E Maintenance therapy for 1–2 years after initial intensive chemotherapy

Question 128

A 30-year-old woman presents with cough and dyspnea on exertion. She has not experienced fever, weight loss or night sweats, but has had increasing pruritus. Chest X-ray reveals a large mediastinal mass and an excisional biopsy is consistent with nodular sclerosis Hodgkin lymphoma. Staging studies reveal small lower cervical lymph nodes, an 11-cm mediastinal mass and splenomegaly. The patient is a nonsmoker, has no other medical problems and has two siblings who are in good health.

Q Which of the following is the most appropriate initial management?

A ABVD for 6–8 cycles
B ABVD for 2–4 cycles and involved field radiation therapy
C MOPP/ABV for 6–8 cycles
D ABVD for 6–8 cycles, followed by radiation to the mediastinum
E MOPP/ABV followed by total nodal irradiation

Question 129

A 5-year-old boy with Diamond–Blackfan anemia undergoes a matched bone marrow transplant from his HLA-matched sibling. He tolerates the chemotherapy and radiation without difficulty and demonstrates neutrophil engraftment by day 15 and is discharged from the hospital. He continues to require platelet transfusions until day 25. Although his PRBC transfusion requirements decrease to every 7 days, he continues to need them at day 40.

Q What is the most likely cause of this patient's condition?

A The patient has HUS–TTP
B Graft failure
C The donor has Diamond–Blackfan anemia
D The patient has developed myelodysplastic syndrome (MDS), an increasing problem post-stem cell transplant
E The patient and donor red cells are of different blood type

Question 130

A 42-year-old male presents to the emergency department with an episode of dizziness. Routine blood chemistry reveals an activated partial thromboplastin time (APTT) >150 s. The laboratory reports that a protamine sulfate neutralization test did not shorten the APTT, but the APTT normalized when a 50 : 50 mix with pooled normal plasma was performed. The patient is well, without any current or previous evidence of bleeding. Although previously unnoticed, his APTT was similarly prolonged at the time of scoliosis surgery 12 years previously. The INR is normal.

Q Which of the following should be performed next to evaluate this patient?

A Measure factor VIII level
B Measure the bleeding time and the von Willebrand antigen level
C Measure factor XIII level
D Measure factor XII level
E A therapeutic trial of vitamin K

Question 131

A 72-year-old man is evaluated for three episodes of acute, severe and symptomatic thrombocytopenia that have occurred in the past 4 weeks. With each episode the patient suddenly developed purpura and epistaxis. He was treated in each case with intravenous methylprednisolone and had a rapid recovery of his platelet count to levels >500,000/μL. The sudden falls in the platelet count occurred despite maintenance prednisone therapy (1 mg/kg/day). He was diagnosed with idiopathic thrombocytopenic purpura (ITP) 12 years ago and required splenectomy; he has not had recurrent thrombocytopenia until these recent episodes. He was taking multiple medications for diabetes and quinine for musculoskeletal symptoms at the time of his first episode of acute thrombocytopenia 1 month ago.

Q What are the most appropriate evaluation and management for this patient?

A Continue prednisone; add rituximab, 375 mg/m^2/week for 4 weeks
B Evaluate for the presence of an accessory spleen
C Suspect lymphoma, order CT scan of chest and abdomen
D Suspect drug-induced thrombocytopenia, unrelated to previously diagnosed ITP
E Suspect thrombotic thrombocytopenic purpura (TTP), plan to evaluate peripheral blood smear and other aspects of microangiopathic hemolysis if thrombocytopenia recurs

Question 132

A 72-year-old man presents to the emergency department with acute-onset shortness of breath and two episodes of hemoptysis. He has known metastatic prostate carcinoma and recently was hospitalized because of a pathological fracture of the femur requiring open reduction and internal fixation. A ventilation perfusion scan demonstrates a segmental mismatched perfusion defect.

Q Which of the following is the most appropriate next step in the management of this patient?

A A contrast-enhanced helical/spiral chest CT scan should be performed
B Ultrasound of the legs
C Treatment with intravenous heparin for 4–6 months
D Treatment with enoxaparin for 4–6 days at a dosage of 30 mg twice daily
E Treatment with dalteparin, 200 U/kg once daily indefinitely

Question 133

You are asked to see a 34-year-old Laotian man because of severe anemia. He underwent an orthotopic liver transplant 17 days earlier for cirrhosis secondary to chronic hepatitis C. His postoperative course was uncomplicated and he received a single unit of packed red blood cell transfusion on the first postoperative day. His physical examination is remarkable for scleral icterus and postoperative scars. A week ago, his hemoglobin was 10.3 g/dL. His hemoglobin is now 6.3 g/dL, his LDH is 643 IU, and his bilirubin is 3.1 mg/dL. A peripheral blood smear reveals polychromasia, occasional spherocytes and rare schistocytes. The patient's blood type is A-positive; the liver donor's blood type is O-positive. The direct antibody test is positive for IgG.

Q What antibodies would be found in the patient's serum and eluate from his red blood cells?

A Anti-Rh antibodies
B Anti-A antibodies
C Red cell panagglutinins
D Cold agglutinins

Question 134

A 33-year-old male with myelodysplastic syndrome has bright red blood in his stool and a platelet count of 22,000/μL. He receives leukoreduced and irradiated platelet concentrates transfused over 20 min. He is known to be group B, Rh-positive but receives group AB, Rh-positive platelets as there are no group B platelets available. Two hours after the transfusion, he develops respiratory distress manifested as dyspnea without stridor or wheezing. His systolic blood pressure drops slightly and his temperature rises to 99.9°F. A pulse oximeter shows 87% saturation and he has bilateral rales on auscultation. He has no urticaria. His electrocardiogram is unchanged.

Q What is the most likely cause of this adverse transfusion reaction?

A Bacterial contamination
B Anaphylaxis
C ABO incompatibility
D Leukoagglutinins
E Circulatory overload

Question 135

A 14-year-old boy was treated at age 12 for orbital retinoblastoma with carboplatin, etoposide, vincristine, doxorubicin and cyclophosphamide. He presents 18 months later with fatigue, epistaxis and easy bruising. His CBC results are: hemoglobin 8.1 g/dL, WBC 17,000/μL with 80% blasts and 12,000/μL platelets. The blasts are butyrate esterase positive.

Q Which of the following cytogenetic abnormalities is most likely associated with this leukemia?

A Balanced translocation involving 11q23
B inv(16) (p13;q22)
C inv(3) (q21;q26)
D t(11;17)(q13;q21)

Question 136

A 38-year-old woman, gravida 3, para 2, is referred in the second trimester of a normal pregnancy for asymptomatic thrombocytopenia. The onset of thrombocytopenia preceded her first pregnancy. In the first trimester of her current pregnancy her platelet count fluctuated between 80,000 and 120,000/μL. In the last 2 weeks it fell to 50,000/μL. In one of her two prior pregnancies, her platelet nadir was 60,000/μL. She does not recall receiving any treatment for thrombocytopenia during or between pregnancies. She had no hemorrhagic complications and delivered two normal infants, neither of whom had neonatal thrombocytopenia. Her spleen is intact. Her history is negative for pathological bleeding, physical examination is remarkable only for signs of pregnancy. The remaining blood cell counts and peripheral blood morphology are normal.

Q Which of the following is/are the most appropriate evaluation(s) and management choice(s)?

A Start prednisone 80 mg/day now and plan to taper when platelets reach 100,000/μL
B Administer intravenous immunoglobulin (IVIG) during the final 2 weeks of pregnancy
C Plan to perform a funipuncture (umbilical cord blood sample) late in pregnancy to determine if a Cesarean section would be appropriate
D Perform frequent maternal platelet counts without other interventions directed at the thrombocytopenia unless the maternal platelet count falls below 50,000/μL or there are signs of maternal hemorrhage

Question 137

Q Which of the following statements about prenatal diagnosis of factor VIII deficiency in an at-risk fetus is true?

A Prenatal diagnosis relies on direct demonstration of a characteristic point mutation in the factor VIII gene
B Prenatal diagnosis is not indicated if the fetus is a male
C Prenatal diagnosis may require linkage analysis of the family
D Prenatal diagnosis requires fetal blood obtained by umbilical blood sampling

Question 138

A 37-year-old male is noted to have pancytopenia after presenting to his primary care physician with fatigue. On examination, pallor is noted. He does not have any lymphadenopathy or splenomegaly. The hemoglobin is 5.5 g/dL, absolute reticulocyte count 16×10^9/L, white cell count 0.9×10^9/L, absolute neutrophil count 0.1×10^9/L and platelet count 15×10^9/L. The bone marrow biopsy is aplastic and the bone marrow aspirate smear reveals hypocellular spicules with no evidence of dysplasia or abnormal cells. Bone marrow cytogenetics is normal.

He has three siblings, one of whom is a complete HLA match.

Q Which of the following is the most appropriate management for this patient?

A Antithymocyte globulin (ATG) 40 mg/kg for 4 days + cyclosporine 12 mg/kg/day
B Matched sibling allogeneic stem cell transplant with cyclophosphamide and ATG as conditioning
C Matched sibling allogeneic stem cell transplant with cyclophosphamide and total body irradiation as conditioning
D Granulocyte colony-stimulating factor and erythropoietin therapy

Question 139

A 26-year-old female patient is sent to you for a second opinion regarding the diagnosis of 'porphyria'. She provides you with no outside records for review. She is of Dutch heritage and has a family history of blistering skin lesions, psychiatric problems and chronic abdominal pain. Since puberty the patient has developed intermittent crampy abdominal pain, occasionally requiring hospital admission and intravenous narcotics. Work-up, including an exploratory laparotomy, is unrevealing. She is otherwise healthy and has no current complaints. Examination is significant for multiple scars on the dorsum of her hands as well as a few fresh painless 2-cm blisters.

Q What is the most likely diagnosis?

A Acute intermittent porphyria (AIP)
B Porphyria cutanea tarda
C Variegate porphyria
D Congenital erythropoietic porphyria

Question 140

A 45-year-old man with HIV infection presents with complaints of fevers, night sweats and increasing exercise intolerance because of fatigue and weakness. He has been taking multidrug antiretroviral treatment including AZT, 3TC and indinivir for 5 years. In recent months, his CD4 count has fallen to <100/μL and his HIV viral load has increased to >100,000 copies/mL. He is not on any other medication.

His laboratory studies show a hemoglobin of 8.0 g/dL, MCV 115 fL, platelet count of 100,000/μL and a normal white blood cell count and differential. A corrected reticulocyte count is 1.0%. He has normal electrolytes, blood urea nitrogen (BUN) and creatinine, as well as a normal LDH and haptoglobin.

Q All of the following may contribute to the patient's hematologic findings *except*:

A Chronic parvovirus B19 infection
B AZT
C *Mycobacterium avium* complex
D Thrombotic thrombocytopenic purpura (TTP)
E Disseminated candidemia

Question 141

A 63-year-old Caucasian man comes to you for evaluation and treatment of severe symptomatic anemia. His prior history is significant for mild anemia, cholelithiasis and hypertension. He recalls no recent illness, but was in contact with his grandson who had a rash and febrile illness approximately 10 days ago. His family history is significant for gallstones in multiple family members. Laboratory data are as follows:

	Current	6 months prior (routine)
HCT	14%	35%
MCV	93 fL	106 fL
Platelet count	197,000/μL	268,000/μL
WBC count	4900/μL	5600/μL
Reticulocyte count (uncorrected)	0.1%	4.8%

The peripheral blood smear reveals a mild to moderate number of spherocytes. Red cell transfusion is started.

Q Which of the following is the most appropriate next step in the evaluation of this patient?

A Osmotic fragility testing
B PCR testing for parvovirus DNA
C Direct antiglobulin test (DAT)
D Bone marrow aspirate and biopsy

Question 142

A 29-year-old man with chronic myeloid leukemia (CML) in chronic phase comes for a second opinion regarding therapy. He was recently diagnosed after routine blood tests and is in otherwise excellent health. On examination, he has mild splenomegaly. His WBC count is 22,000/μL with a predominance of maturing myeloid cells. Cytogenetics demonstrated the t(9;22) translocation. He has three siblings, one of whom is a complete HLA match.

Q Which of the following statements is true regarding the therapeutic options for this patient?

A Successful allogeneic transplantation extends the chronic phase of CML, delaying progression to blast crisis
B Successful allogeneic transplantation and a complete hematologic response to imatinib mesylate have a similar probability of long-term disease-free survival
C Successful allogeneic transplantation for this patient with a matched related donor offers >60% chance of cure
D Nonmyeloablative transplant results in higher cure rates than myeloablative transplantation

Question 143

A 19-month-old boy is brought to his pediatrician for evaluation of a progressive skin rash and a protuberant abdomen. His parents also describe decreased activity over the past 2–3 weeks without fever or other systemic signs. Physical examination reveals multiple café au lait macules on the trunk and extremities and a diffuse erythematous rash without petechiae. The liver edge is palpated 4 cm below the right costal margin and the spleen is massively enlarged with extension into the pelvis and across the midline. A CBC shows WBC 22,600/μL with an absolute monocyte count of 5000/μL, hemoglobin 8.1 g/dL and a platelet count of 49,000/μL. The bone marrow is hypercellular with <5% blasts and an expanded number of myelomonocytic cells.

Q Which of the following statements is correct about this patient's condition and its management?

A It occurs primarily in girls
B Fanconi anemia is associated with an increased risk for this disease
C Cell culture and cytogenetic studies are not helpful in diagnosis
D This entity is unique and is not classified with any myeloid malignancy that occurs in adults
E Combination chemotherapy is largely ineffective and allogeneic hematopoietic stem cell transplantation is the treatment of choice

Question 144

A 57-year-old woman with a history of breast cancer, treated with CAF chemotherapy in the past, develops shortness of breath and fatigue. She is found to be profoundly pancytopenic, with a white blood cell count of 1200/μL, hemoglobin of 7.8 g/dL and a platelet count of 23,000/μL. A bone marrow aspirate and biopsy reveal acute myeloid leukemia. The blast cells appear to have a monocytoid appearance. The cytogenetic analysis shows the presence of a chromosome translocation involving chromosome band 11q23, and molecular studies show rearrangement of the MLL gene.

Q Which of the following is the most appropriate therapy for this patient?

A Induction chemotherapy with daunorubicin and cytarabine, followed by one course of high-dose cytarabine, then autologous stem cell transplantation
B Induction chemotherapy with daunorubicin and cytarabine, followed by one course of high-dose cytarabine, then a fully ablative matched related donor allogeneic stem cell transplant
C Induction with daunorubicin and cytarabine, followed by four courses of high-dose cytarabine, then a nonmyeloablative matched unrelated donor transplant
D Induction chemotherapy with daunorubicin and cytarabine, followed by one course of high-dose cytarabine, then a fully ablative matched unrelated donor transplant
E Induction with daunorubicin and cytarabine, followed by one course of high-dose cytarabine, then an autologous stem cell transplant, followed by a nonmyeloablative matched related donor allogeneic stem cell transplant

Question 145

Q Which of the following findings indicates the poorest prognosis in a patient with multiple myeloma?

A Bone marrow plasmacytosis of 35%
B Deletion of the long arm of chromosome 13
C Presence of anemia
D Diffuse lytic bone disease
E Creatinine of 2.8 mg/dL

Question 146

A 3-year-old boy diagnosed with AML obtains a remission with timed intensive chemotherapy. His parents have stored all of the children's cord blood in a private cord blood bank. He has a 3-year-old brother and a 5-year-old sister. On evaluation of the typing, his brother is found to be genotypically identical and his sister is haplo-identical.

Q Which of the following is the most appropriate next therapy for this patient?

A An autologous transplant for consolidation chemotherapy
B A cord blood transplant using his brother's cord blood
C Continued standard chemotherapy and transplant if there is relapse of AML
D Allogeneic transplant using his sister as the donor
E Allogeneic transplant using his brother as the donor

Question 147

Q Which of the following therapies has been shown to reduce the mortality rate in patients with severe sepsis?

A Heparin
B Recombinant tissue factor pathway inhibitor (TFPI)
C Recombinant antithrombin (AT)
D Recombinant activated protein C (rAPC)
E Streptokinase

Question 148

A previously healthy 37-year-old male fractures his tibial plateau through hyperextension while jogging downhill, and has it surgically repaired that day. Two units of nonleukoreduced packed red cells are ordered after surgery for replacement of blood loss through the drain. He has never been transfused before. Thirty minutes into transfusion of the first unit, he has a shaking chill and develops a new fever to 39.5°C accompanied by tachycardia and tachypnea without oxygen desaturation. His blood pressure rises slightly. He denies back or flank pain, and his Foley catheter shows yellow urine. The direct antiglobulin test on a post-transfusion sample is negative.

Q What is the most likely cause of his transfusion reaction?

A Bacterial contamination
B Anaphylaxis
C Incompatibility
D Leukoagglutinins
E Donor-derived cytokines

Question 149

Q Hyperlipidemia impacts the measurement of which of the following components of an automated complete blood count?

A The total red cell count
B The mean platelet volume
C The hemoglobin
D The mean corpuscular volume of erythrocytes

Question 150

A hospital consultation is requested because of thrombocytopenia in an 18-year-old gravida 1, para 0, African-American woman with type 1 diabetes mellitus, in her 29th week of pregnancy. She complains of headache and right upper quadrant pain, but not abnormal bleeding. Her blood pressure is 155/105 mmHg and physical examination shows moderate pitting ankle edema and a normal uterine size for dates with no evidence of hemorrhage. Her abdominal examination is negative. Her hemoglobin is 8.6 g/dL, she has one schistocyte per five high-power fields, platelets are 48,000/μL; urine is 2+ for protein and creatinine is 2.1 mg/dL. Total bilirubin is 3.1 mg/dL, 1.5 mg/dL direct; aspartate transaminase (AST) is 100 (ULN = 40). LDH, PT, PTT and fibrinogen are normal.

Q Which of the following is the most appropriate next step in the management of this patient?

A Plasma exchange
B Magnesium sulfate
C Octreotide and midodrine
D Ultrasonography of the abdomen and pelvis

Question 151

A 53-year-old male complains of discolored urine, especially during the initial urination in the morning. He is not taking any medications. On examination, pallor is noted. There is no lymphadenopathy or splenomegaly. His urine is positive for hemosiderin. The hemoglobin is 7.2 g/dL, absolute reticulocyte count 35×10^9/L, white cell count 2.8×10^9/L, absolute neutrophil count 1.0×10^9/L and platelet count 35×10^9/L. The peripheral smear shows macrocytic red blood cells. The bone marrow biopsy demonstrates 10% cellularity; the bone marrow spicules are hypocellular with mostly lymphocytes and plasma cells. There are very few myeloid or erythroid elements to evaluate but mild erythroid dysplasia can be appreciated. Flow cytometric analysis of blood neutrophils shows decreased expression of CD55 and CD59. A cytogenetic analysis of bone marrow is normal. One of the patient's siblings is a complete HLA match.

Q Which of the following is the most appropriate therapy for this patient?

A Antithymocyte globulin + cyclosporine
B Matched sibling allogeneic stem cell transplant
C Anticoagulation with warfarin
D Prednisone and anticoagulation with coumarin

Question 152

A 43-year-old construction worker is referred to you for evaluation of blistering skin lesions over his arms and hands. He wears short-sleeved shirts and spends much of the day working in the sun. His medical history is significant only for previous intravenous drug use. He takes no medications and consumes two to three beers each day. Physical examination is significant for multiple well-healed skin lesions over his hands and arms. A few fresh blisters are noted over his hands bilaterally. A complete blood count is normal. Iron studies are shown below (reference values in parentheses):

Serum iron	195 μg/dL (normal, 42–135 μg/dL)
Serum total iron-binding capacity	389 μg/dL (normal, 225–430 μg/dL)
Transferrin saturation	51% (normal, 20–50%)
Serum ferritin	632 ng/mL (normal, 30–400 ng/mL)

Q Which of the following is most appropriate in further evaluating this patient?

A Urine studies for porphobilinogen (PBG) and δ-aminolevulinic acid (ALA)
B Liver function tests and hepatitis serologies
C Red cell enzyme levels of PBG deaminase
D Hemochromatosis genetic testing in all of his children

Question 153

A 30-year-old man received an allogeneic bone marrow transplantation from an ABO-mismatched HLA-identical sibling for the treatment of chronic myeloid leukemia. Six months following engraftment the patient continues to require RBC transfusions for severe normocytic anemia. White blood cells and platelets are within normal limits. A bone marrow examination shows markedly reduced red cell precursors.

Q The most likely etiology of the persistent anemia is:

A Immunosuppression-induced anemia
B Persistent leukemia
C Evolving aplastic anemia
D Red cell aplasia resulting from ABO isohemagglutinins

Question 154

A previously healthy 63-year-old man complains of a 2-month history of fever, chills and night sweats. He has lost 10 lb during this period. More recently he has developed chest pain, shortness of breath and fatigue. He is admitted with acute substernal chest pain that is refractory to standard treatment for angina. ST depression is sustained on repeated electrocardiograms.

He has received 8 units of packed red blood cells in the last month, including two this morning without a sustained increase in the hematocrit. Laboratory data and peripheral blood smear (see Figure) are shown below:

Hematocrit	21%
MCV	143 fL
WBC count	4900/μL
Platelet count	145,000/μL
Reticulocyte count	6.1%
LDH	1449 U/L

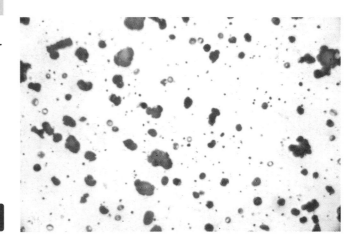

Q After hemodynamic stabilization, which of the following should be initiated as initial treatment?

A Cytotoxic chemotherapy
B Prednisone

C Plasma exchange therapy using a blood-warming device
D Splenectomy
E Standard transfusion of two more units of blood

D Allogeneic stem cell transplantation is the treatment of choice if a suitable donor is found

Question 155

A 55-year-old woman with recurrent headaches presents for evaluation. Her primary care physician drew a CBC that demonstrated a WBC count of 24,000/μL. Her headaches have been long-standing and respond to sumatriptan. A CBC from 6 months ago showed a WBC count of 22,000/μL. She denies weakness, easy bruising or bleeding; she has no history of thrombosis. On physical examination, her spleen is palpable 4 cm below the costal margin. Review of the blood smear shows basophilia, metamyelocytes and myelocytes. Peripheral blood cytogenetics is negative for the t(9;22) translocation.

Q What is the most appropriate next step in the management of this patient?

A Empiric antibiotic therapy
B Determination of leukocyte alkaline phosphatase (LAP) score
C Re-evaluate in 3 months
D PCR for the *BCR-ABL* fusion gene

Question 156

A healthy 9-year-old girl has a routine yearly CBC performed in the cancer follow-up clinic. This shows a WBC count of 2400/μL, hemoglobin 8.6 g/dL and platelets 109,000/μL. The history is remarkable for successful treatment of an embryonal rhabdomyosarcoma of the jaw between ages 3 and 5 years. Her therapy included surgery, involved field radiation and combination chemotherapy with high-dose alkylating agents and other drugs. Her physical examination today is unremarkable. The bone marrow is mildly hypocellular with <5% blasts and moderate trilineage dysplasia.

Q Which of the following statements about this patient's disorder is true?

A The pancytopenia is unlikely to be related to her previous cancer treatment
B Her bone marrow is likely to show a translocation involving chromosome band 11q23
C Intensive induction chemotherapy is indicated at this time

Question 157

A 26-year-old medical student presents with fatigue and easy bruising. She is found to have profound pancytopenia and a bone marrow study establishes the diagnosis of acute promyelocytic leukemia. Cytogenetic studies show the t(15;17) translocation; molecular genetic studies further confirm the diagnosis by presence of the PML-RARα fusion protein. She is induced into remission uneventfully with a combination of all-*trans* retinoic acid (ATRA) plus daunorubicin and cytarabine. She receives two courses of consolidation chemotherapy with daunorubicin alone for 3 days each, and her subsequent cytogenetic and molecular studies are negative.

Q Which of the following would be appropriate therapy for this patient?

A Maintenance therapy with all-*trans* retinoic acid (ATRA), plus low-dose chemotherapy (6-mercaptopurine and methotrexate) for 2 years
B ATRA, plus low-dose chemotherapy (6-mercaptopurine and methotrexate) for 5 years
C Maintenance with ATRA, plus arsenic trioxide for four courses
D Autologous stem cell transplantation
E Maintenance therapy with ATRA, plus low-dose chemotherapy (6-mercaptopurine plus methotrexate) for 1 year, followed by autologous stem cell transplantation

Question 158

A 28-year-old woman presents for follow-up after recently moving to the area. She was treated for stage IIA nodular sclerosing Hodgkin lymphoma at age 19 years with mantle and periaortic radiation therapy. She has been feeling well and is hoping to start a family.

Q Which of the following would be the most appropriate follow-up for this patient?

A PET scan to evaluate for residual disease
B Yearly CT scan of the chest, abdomen and pelvis
C Yearly complete blood count
D Monthly breast examinations with mammograms starting next year
E Routine health maintenance as for other women of her age

Question 159

A 56-year-old man undergoes coronary angiography. Seven days later he presents to the emergency department with an acute myocardial infarction, despite having normal coronary arteries on angiography. His ECG demonstrates ST segment elevation and he undergoes primary percutaneous coronary intervention (PCI). Two days later he develops left leg ischemia which requires surgical embolectomy of a superior femoral artery (SFA) thrombus. His blood tests demonstrate a white blood cell count of 4.5, hemoglobin of 12.3 g/dL and platelet count of 160/μL. His history is unremarkable except for a traumatic splenectomy at age 16 years.

Q Which of the following is the most appropriate immediate management for this patient?

A Intravenous heparin, followed by warfarin to achieve an INR of 2.0–3.0, for a minimum of 6 months
B Subcutaneous low-molecular-weight heparin (LMWH), followed by warfarin to achieve an INR of 2.0–3.0, for a minimum of 6 months
C Lepirudin, followed by warfarin to achieve an INR of 2.0–3.0, for a minimum of 6 months
D tPA, followed by intravenous heparin and warfarin to achieve an INR of 2.0–3.0, for a minimum of 6 months
E Warfarin alone; use of a parenteral anticoagulant might worsen the thrombosis

Question 160

A 30-year-old male with newly diagnosed AML had an admission platelet count of 17,000/μL. He received four pooled platelet concentrates for placement of a PICC line, with a post-transfusion platelet count of 52,000/μL at 1 h. His platelet count was 47,000/μL the following morning and 37,000/μL the next day. He has no fever, organomegaly or history of bleeding and is not on antibiotics. He has no petechiae, purpura or other signs of hemorrhage. His stool is negative for occult blood and his PT and APTT are normal.

Q When should you order his next prophylactic platelet transfusion?

A Platelet count below 30,000
B Platelet count below 25,000
C Platelet count below 20,000
D Platelet count below 15,000

Question 161

A 40-year-old man is referred for evaluation of cervical adenopathy. On examination, the left anterior cervical node measures 3 × 4 cm. A biopsy of the node is obtained. The referring physician obtained CT scans of the chest, abdomen and pelvis, which were normal. The bone marrow biopsy is negative for lymphoma. The flow cytometry results on the lymph node reveal that the tumour cells are CD20, CD45, BCL6, EMA and IgG kappa positive and CD10, CD5, CD15 and CD30 negative.

Q Which of the following is the most likely diagnosis?

A Mantle cell lymphoma
B Follicular lymphoma
C Nodular lymphocyte-predominant Hodgkin lymphoma
D Lymphocyte-rich classic Hodgkin lymphoma

Question 162

A 35-year-old pregnant Chinese woman asks about thrombophilia as a risk for having a spontaneous abortion, because a previous pregnancy spontaneously terminated after 11 weeks. She is gravida 2, para 0 and in the middle of her first trimester. She has no personal history of venous thromboembolic (VTE) disease. No diagnostic tests for thrombophilia have been performed on the patient or her family members.

Q Which one of the following presents the highest risk for spontaneous abortion and fetal death in this patient?

A Antiphospholipid syndrome
B Heterozygous factor V Leiden
C Protein C deficiency
D Antithrombin III deficiency

Question 163

A 16-year-old female presents with fatigue and increasing shortness of breath noted when she plays basketball. These symptoms are similar to those she experienced 6 years ago when she was diagnosed with severe aplastic anemia. At that time, she was treated with antithymocyte globulin and cyclosporine with a good response. She does not have any siblings.

On examination, pallor is noted. The remainder of her physical examination is normal. The hemoglobin is 6.5 g/dL, absolute reticulocyte count 15×10^9/L, white cell count 2.8×10^9/L, absolute neutrophil count 1.0×10^9/L and platelet count 35×10^9/L. A bone biopsy shows cellularity varying from 10% to 30%. On the aspirate smears, megaloblastic erythroid forms and small megakaryocytes with unilobed nuclei are noted. There are <5% myeloblasts.

Q (a) The most likely cytogenetic abnormality on a marrow aspirate specimen is:

A t(8;21)
B t(4;11)
C inv16
D Monosomy 7
E Monosomy 8

Q (b) The most appropriate treatment strategy for the above patient with a cytogenetic abnormality is:

A Induction and consolidation chemotherapy
B Immunosuppression with antithymocyte globulin and cyclosporine
C Matched unrelated donor stem cell transplantation
D Erythropoietin and granulocyte colony-stimulating factor (G-CSF) only

Question 164

A 35-year-old woman with sickle cell disease and HIV-1 infection presents to the emergency room with complaints of severe weakness and dyspnea increasing over the previous 2–3 weeks. Her HIV infection is asymptomatic—an HIV viral load was undetectable and CD4 count was 400/μL 1 week ago. Her only medication is daily folate. Her 4-year-old son, who is currently in good health, was noted to have a transient fever and rash 1 month ago.

Her laboratory tests in the emergency room show a hemoglobin of 3.0 g/dL, MCV 88 fL, platelets 150,000/μL, a WBC count of 20,000/μL and a corrected reticulocyte count of 0.9%.

Q In addition to red cell transfusions, which of the following interventions is the most likely to help in treating this patient's anemia?

A Intravenous gammaglobulin therapy
B Institution of AZT monotherapy
C Interferon-α and ribavirin therapy
D Trimethoprim-sulfamethoxazole
E Splenectomy

Question 165

A 45-year-old man is referred to your office with fatigue, lethargy and exertional dyspnea. His hematocrit is 24%. Past history is significant for a prosthetic aortic valve placed 8 years ago because of complications of rheumatic heart disease. Current medications include warfarin and an over-the-counter decongestant.

On physical examination, the patient is well appearing, has mild scleral icterus and a grade 3–6 systolic ejection murmur heard best at the left upper sternal border with radiation to the neck. An echocardiogram reveals a perivalvular leak, turbulent flow and a left ventricular ejection fraction of 54%. Laboratory data are as follows:

Hematocrit	29%
MCV	79 fL
Platelet count	198,000/μL
Leukocyte count	5600/μL
Red cell distribution width	17.1%
Reticulocyte count	10.5%

Q On review of the peripheral blood smear, you are most likely to find:

A Schistocytes
B Bite cells
C Spherocytes
D Stomatocytes

Question 166

A 32-year-old patient is transferred to your hospital with fever and WBC count of 40,000/μL, 80% of which are blasts. Flow cytometry immunophenotypic analysis reveals that the blasts are $CD13^+$, $CD19^-$ and $CD33^+$. Cytogenetics reveals the presence of the t(9;22) translocation. He has four siblings.

Q The most appropriate treatment plan would be:

A Induction chemotherapy with an anthracycline and cytarabine followed by an autologous stem cell transplant
B Induction chemotherapy with an anthracycline and cytarabine followed by four cycles of high-dose cytarabine

C Imatinib mesylate with the addition of interferon-α if the patient fails to respond or relapses on imatinib alone
D Induction chemotherapy followed by a matched related or unrelated donor stem cell transplant, if possible

Question 167

A 68-year-old man with AML presents in first relapse after a first remission duration of 13 months.

Q Which of the following would be the best reinduction strategy?

A Daunorubicin plus high-dose cytarabine
B High-dose cytarabine plus gemtuzumab ozogamicin
C Daunorubicin plus gemtuzumab ozogamicin
D Gemtuzumab ozogamicin
E Daunorubicin plus cytarabine and gemtuzumab ozogamicin

Question 168

A 68-year-old African-American man with a history of multiple myeloma presents with increasing fatigue and back pain. He is found to have progressive lytic lesions and an IgG kappa monoclonal spike of 3.8 g/dL. He was initially treated with VAD (vincristine, doxorubicin and dexamethasone) followed by an autologous stem cell transplant with an excellent response. After relapsing 6 months ago, he had a brief response to thalidomide but is now progressing.

Q Which of the following would be the most appropriate therapy for this patient?

A Repeat high-dose therapy with autologous stem cell rescue
B Palliative care
C Melphalan and prednisone
D Bortezomib
E Zoledronic acid

Question 169

A 70-year-old man is to undergo elective total hip joint replacement. He is diabetic, has poorly controlled hypertension and has had a stroke secondary to atrial fibrillation within the last 3 months. He takes warfarin for secondary prevention of recurrent thrombosis. Although advised to defer surgery for several months given his recent stroke, the patient insists on surgery because he is severely disabled by hip pain.

Q Around the time of surgery, which strategy should be used to manage warfarin therapy?

A Warfarin should be withheld for 72 h and restarted immediately after surgery
B Warfarin should be withheld for 5 days, and the patient admitted to the hospital for intravenous unfractionated heparin 5000 U subcutaneously twice daily 3 days preoperatively. Warfarin should be restarted in the immediate postoperative period
C Warfarin should be withheld for 5 days, and the patient should receive enoxaparin 30 mg/day subcutaneously beginning 3 days prior to the surgery. Warfarin should be restarted in the immediate postoperative period
D Warfarin should be withheld for 5 days, and the patient should receive enoxaparin 1 mg/kg subcutaneously twice daily beginning 3 days prior to the procedure. Warfarin should be restarted in the immediate postoperative period
E Withholding warfarin is too risky given the recent stroke; the patient should continue on warfarin throughout the perioperative period. The surgeon and hematologist must ensure the INR does not fall below 2.0

Question 170

A 6-month-old, group A, Rh-positive male weighing 8.5 kg had cranioplasty for complex craniosynostosis and was sent to the neurosurgical intensive care unit for postoperative care. There was minimal bleeding during surgery but the hemoglobin dropped from 12.0 to 8.5 g/dL over the following 24 h from subgaleal hemorrhage. The vital signs were stable, and the heart rate and blood pressure were normal for an infant of this age. A unit of packed red blood cells, collected as a directed donation from the infant's group O, Rh-positive father, was transfused over 1 h. At the end of the transfusion, tachycardia was noted, along with hypertension and respiratory distress and dusky skin. No fever, red urine, hives or mucosal edema was noted.

Q What is the most likely cause of the transfusion reaction?

A Bacterial contamination
B Anaphylaxis
C ABO incompatibility

D Leukoagglutinins
E Circulatory overload

Question 171

A 28-year-old man is referred to your office with a diagnosis of acute leukemia. His hemoglobin is 8.2 g/dL, his WBC count is 84,400/μL and his platelet count is 17,000/μL. The peripheral blood blast nuclei have a bilobed appearance. The bone marrow contains >80% blasts. Rare cytoplasmic granules are present on the Romanowsky stain. Myeloperoxidase is positive, butyrate esterase is negative. The blasts are CD33 and CD2 positive, and CD34, HLA-DR, CD15, glycophorin and CD61 negative. Cytogenetic studies are obtained.

Q Which of the following cytogenetic abnormalities is most likely in this patient?

A t(8;16)(p11;p13)
B t(8;21)(q22;q22)
C t(15;17)(q22;q12)
D t(1;22)(p13;q13)

Question 172

A 63-year-old businessman is referred with thrombocytopenia. His platelet count has fallen over the past 6 weeks. Other hematologic studies and review of his peripheral blood film are normal. He was seen in hematology consultation 2 years previously. At that time his platelet count was 90,000/μL. He has never received treatment for thrombocytopenia. At the time of the current consultation, a platelet count on a fresh heparinized sample is 70,000/μL. WBC, hemoglobin and hematocrit are normal. Peripheral blood morphology is also normal. He reports that he has bled from shaving cuts for 5–10 min on two occasions and has noticed two unexplained bruises on his right arm during the past 3 months. Otherwise, history and physical examination, including a complete list of medications and exposures, are unrevealing.

Q Which of the following is the most appropriate management of this patient?

A Antiplatelet antibody and fluorescence antinuclear antibody test
B CT scans of the chest and abdomen
C Bone marrow examination
D Periodic measurement of platelet counts

Question 173

You are asked to evaluate a newborn male on day 2 of life because he has had persistent bleeding for 2 h following a circumcision. The physical examination is otherwise normal. The pregnancy was uncomplicated. The hemoglobin, white blood cell count and platelet count are normal. You obtain a family history of another male relative who may have a bleeding disorder.

Q Which is the most effective step to take next in the management of this patient?

A Apply direct pressure to the weeping surgical site
B Administer recombinant factor VIII preparation
C Treat with cryoprecipitate
D Transfuse fresh frozen plasma

Question 174

Q In a patient preparing to undergo autologous stem cell transplantation, CD34^{+} cell counts can guide the timing of stem cell collection for which of the following reasons?

A CD34^{+} cell counts correlate with colony-forming unit–granulocyte macrophage (CFU-GM) numbers
B CD34^{+} cell counts correlate with marrow repopulating potential
C CD34^{+} cell counts correlate with progenitor (or transit amplifying cell) characteristics
D All of the above

Question 175

A 14-year-old boy presents with 2 days of extreme malaise and jaundice. Two weeks ago he developed a nonproductive cough, malaise and fever. He was prescribed azithromycin and respiratory symptoms have since resolved. He has no significant past medical history and takes no medications on a routine basis. On physical examination, he is afebrile, respiratory rate is 18 and heart rate is 106 and regular. He appears pale. Scleral icterus and jaundice are noted. No lymphadenopathy or hepatosplenomegaly is appreciated. Laboratory data reveal the following:

Hematocrit	24%
Platelet count	356,000/μL
Leukocyte count	4600/μL
MCV	144 fL
Red cell distribution width	16.1%
Reticulocyte count (uncorrected)	12%

Review of the peripheral blood smear is requested and a direct antiglobulin test (DAT, Coombs) is ordered.

Q Which of the following combinations of direct antiglobulin test (DAT, Coombs test) results and red cell morphology are most likely in this patient?

	Coombs test		
	IgG	Complement	Red cell morphology
A	+	–	Agglutination
B	–	+	Spherocytes
C	–	+	Agglutination
D	+	–	Spherocytes

Question 176

A 2-year-old boy with Down syndrome presents with petechiae. He had a transient myeloproliferative disorder (TMPD) in the newborn period. Physical examination shows hepatosplenomegaly and adenopathy. Laboratory data include: hemoglobin 8.5 g/dL, WBC 35,000/μL (67% blasts) and platelets 45,000/μL.

Q The most likely diagnosis is:

A B-precursor acute lymphocytic leukemia
B Burkitt leukemia
C Acute promyelocytic leukemia (M3)
D Megakaryocytic leukemia (M7)
E Recurrent TMPD

Question 177

A 72-year-old man presents for evaluation of worsening anemia. He has had progressive renal insufficiency over the last several months which has been attributed to his long history of hypertension and diabetes mellitus. Physical examination reveals mild hepatomegaly and 1+ lower extremity edema. Laboratory data include a hemoglobin of 8.9 g/dL, creatinine 2.8 g/dL and an IgG lambda monoclonal protein of 0.8 g/dL. Urinalysis is significant for 3+ protein and a 24-h urine protein is 6.2 g/dL.

Q Which of the following is most appropriate at this time?

A Bone marrow biopsy
B Renal biopsy
C Plasma exchange
D Erythropoietin injections three times weekly
E Liver biopsy

Question 178

A 2-week-old, group A, Rh-negative premature male, gestational age 28 weeks, has anemia of prematurity. He is on gavage feeding, and requires periodic red cell transfusion to replace blood lost for laboratory testing. His mother is group O, Rh-positive, and is known to be HIV-seropositive but CMV-seronegative. Her antibody screen was negative at delivery.

Q Which of the following transfusion-related complications is most likely to be prevented by using leukocyte-reduced blood in this infant?

A CMV infection
B Alloimmunization
C Graft-versus-host disease
D Febrile nonhemolytic reactions
E Hemolytic reactions

Question 179

A 16-year-old, 60-kg boy with homozygous sickle cell disease (Hb SS) is admitted for laparoscopic cholecystectomy indicated as treatment for symptomatic gallstones. The hemoglobin level the day prior to admission was 8.0 g/dL.

Q Which of the following is the most appropriate perioperative prophylaxis for this patient?

A Perform single volume exchange transfusion prior to surgery
B Transfuse two units packed red blood cells prior to surgery
C Maintain blood oxygen saturation >95% during anesthesia
D Begin hydroxyurea 3 days prior to surgery

Question 180

A 17-year-old female college freshman has recently moved to the area and is referred to you for follow-up of a congenital anemia. She is unaware of the name of the disorder but recalls a history of multiple red blood cell transfusions during childhood. She underwent splenectomy at age 12 years and has not required RBC transfusion since the surgery. Her development has been normal and she carries out daily activities and participates in intramural sports without marked fatigue. Laboratory data are as follows:

Hemoglobin	8.6 g/dL
Hematocrit	26%
MCV	113 fL
WBC count	13,800/μL
Platelet count	556,000/μL
Reticulocyte count	26%

Peripheral smear is shown below.

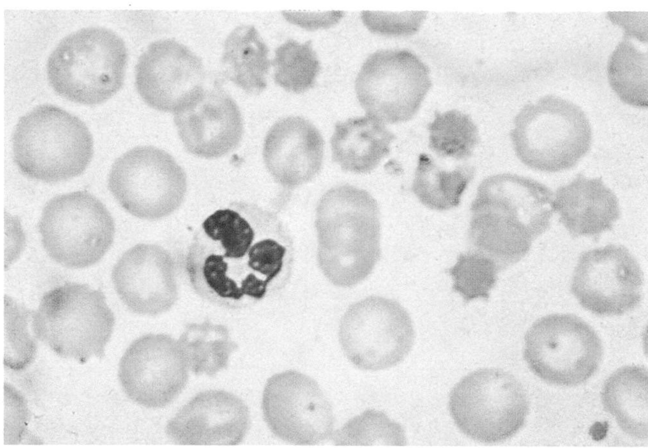

Q The laboratory test most likely to lead to the correct diagnosis is:

A Pyrimidine-5′-nucleotidase activity
B Hemoglobin electrophoresis
C G6PD level
D Direct antiglobulin test (DAT, Coombs test)
E Pyruvate kinase activity

Question 181

A 10-year-old male develops proptosis of his left eye. Physical examination shows no organomegaly or adenopathy. CT scan shows a posterior intraorbital mass with minimal erosion of bone. A CBC is normal. A bone marrow biopsy shows 5% myeloblasts. Biopsy of the mass is compatible with granulocytic sarcoma (chloroma).

Q Which of the following is the most appropriate therapy for this patient?

A Irradiation
B Chemotherapy as for AML
C Chemotherapy as for ALL
D Chemotherapy for AML plus irradiation
E Chemotherapy for ALL plus irradiation

Question 182

A 72-year-old woman returns for follow-up of her monoclonal gammopathy of undetermined significance (MGUS). She continues to feel well and has a normal chemistry panel and CBC. Her serum protein electrophoresis confirms an IgG kappa monoclonal spike of 1.2 g/dL, up from 0.8 g/dL 1 year ago. Bone marrow biopsy reveals 4% plasma cells and her skeletal survey is normal.

Q Which of the following is most appropriate at this time?

A Melphalan and prednisone
B No further therapy or work-up is necessary
C Dexamethasone pulses
D Low-dose thalidomide
E Periodic monitoring of protein, blood counts and skeletal survey

Question 183

A term, well infant is born without complications after a normal pregnancy and initial nursery stay. Upon drawing the metabolic screen, the baby is noted to have prolonged oozing from the heelstick sample. CBC, platelet count, PT, APTT and fibrinogen were normal. Family history is negative. He returns for the 2-week check and the mother notices that the umbilical cord has been oozing for 4 days. A screening test for factor XIII deficiency is ordered and the baby's clot does not dissolve in 5 M urea. The euglobulin lysis time (ELT) was <1 h.

Q The most likely diagnosis is:

A Heterozygous factor XIII deficiency
B Homozygous antiplasmin deficiency
C Mild hemophilia B (factor IX deficiency)
D von Willebrand disease
E Tissue plasminogen activator (TPA) excess

Question 184

A 45-year-old woman presents for outpatient assessment. She had deep vein thrombosis at the age of 25 years while taking the oral contraceptive pill. Since then she has had two unremarkable pregnancies. She is planning to undergo reconstructive surgery on her left knee; this procedure will require her to be in a full leg cast for 6 weeks postoperatively. An uncle and her maternal grandmother had pulmonary embolism after orthopedic surgery. The patient has been tested by her primary care physician and was found to be heterozygous for the factor V Leiden mutation.

Q What perioperative management strategy is most appropriate?

A No antithrombotic prophylaxis
B Warfarin administered to achieve an INR of 2.0–3.0 for the duration of her immobilization
C Hospitalization for the duration of her immobilization and intravenous unfractionated heparin guided by her activated partial thromboplastin time (APTT)
D Therapeutic doses of enoxaparin for the duration of her immobilization
E Given her high risk of thrombosis, she should not undergo surgery

Question 185

An 18-hour-old black female is noted to be jaundiced. Pregnancy, labor and delivery were normal. There is no family history of anemia or jaundice. Physical examination is otherwise normal. The hemoglobin is 12.0 g/dL, hematocrit 37%, MCV 90 fL and reticulocyte count 16%. The WBC and platelet counts are normal. The peripheral blood smear is shown below (see Figure). The baby and mother are both blood group O-positive. The direct antiglobulin test is negative.

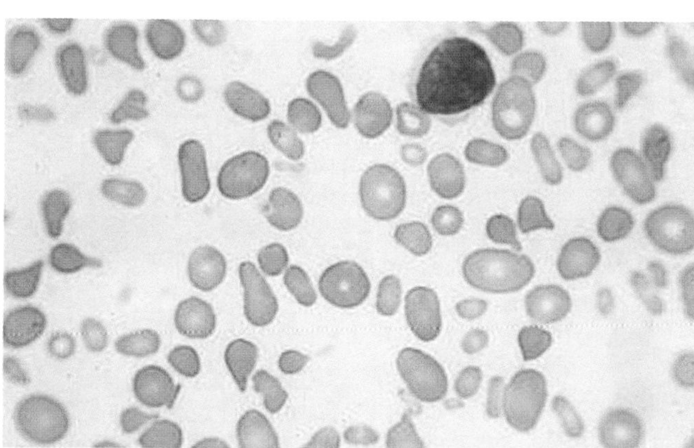

Q Which of the following causes of hereditary hemolytic anemia is most likely in this infant?

A Sickle cell anemia
B Hereditary elliptocytosis
C G6PD deficiency
D α Thalassemia
E β Thalassemia

Question 186

A 4-year-old girl is diagnosed with M2 AML. Her initial WBC is 25,000/μL. The leukemia cell karyotype is normal. She is in remission after two courses of timed intensive chemotherapy.

Q Which of the following is the optimal treatment for this patient?

A Chemotherapy
B Chemotherapy plus cranial irradiation
C Autologous stem cell transplantation
D Matched sibling stem cell transplantation
E Unrelated donor stem cell transplantation

Question 187

A 29-year-old man has a history of stage IVB mixed cellularity Hodgkin lymphoma, treated with eight cycles of ABVD. He presents for evaluation of recurring night sweats 11 months after completing his therapy. Physical examination is significant for palpable splenomegaly and CT scans reveal retroperitoneal adenopathy. Lymph node biopsy confirms recurrent Hodgkin lymphoma and a bone marrow biopsy is positive.

Q The most appropriate therapy for this patient is:

A Matched sibling allogeneic stem cell transplant
B Referral for high-dose therapy with autologous stem cell transplant
C MOPP chemotherapy for 6–8 cycles
D ABVD chemotherapy for 6–8 cycles
E Involved field radiation therapy

Question 188

A 5-year-old female has recurrent streptococcal pharyngitis and enlarged tonsils. Her pediatrician consults with an ENT surgeon who recommends tonsillectomy and adenoidectomy. She comes to see you for a preoperative assessment. History reveals a recent streptococcal infection 1 week ago; she is still on penicillin. Family history confirms normal maternal menses lasting 4–5 days (changing pads four times daily). The patient has nosebleeds, 1–2 times monthly during the winter season, which stop with pressure. Laboratory tests reveal normal CBC and platelet count, PT 12 s, APTT 48 s (10 s prolonged), fibrinogen 200 mg/dL; 1 : 1 mixing studies of the APTT show little correction (immediately and at 1 h) to 46 s.

Q What is the best way to confirm your suspected diagnosis?

A Obtain a more detailed family bleeding history
B Repeat the APTT
C Perform a phospholipid neutralization of the APTT
D Perform factor VIII, IX and XI assays

Question 189

You are called by the emergency room attending physician to evaluate a 2-year-old child noted to have a platelet count of 100×10^9/L and red cell fragments (schistocytes) reported on the peripheral blood smear. This patient has a history of gastroenteritis and diarrhea of 1 week's duration. Other laboratory results include a total bilirubin level of 2.5 mg/dL, blood urea nitrogen of 40 mg/dL and creatinine of 22.1 mg/dL. You admit the patient to the hospital.

Q Which of the following is the most appropriate management step to take next with this patient?

A Obtain a stool culture
B Administer fresh frozen plasma
C Begin plasmapheresis
D Start aspirin and dipyridamole

Question 190

A 7-year-old girl with hemoglobin SC disease presents with low-grade fever, pain in both legs, and swelling and tenderness over the proximal right tibia. Hemoglobin is 10.0 g/dL, hematocrit 31%, reticulocyte count 3.8% and WBC count 17,000/μL with 66% neutrophils, 2% bands and the remainder lymphocytes and monocytes.

Q Which of the following is the best strategy for management of this patient?

A Analgesic therapy
B Antibiotic therapy
C Splinting of the right tibia
D Orthopedic consultation for bone aspiration and biopsy

Question 191

A 10-year-old boy with M2 AML relapses in his bone marrow 8 months after diagnosis, 2 months after completing intensive chemotherapy. He enters a second remission with cytosine arabinoside plus daunorubicin.

Q Which of the following is the most appropriate therapy for this patient?

A Monoclonal antibody
B High-dose cytosine arabinoside
C Farnesyl transferase inhibitor
D Autologous stem cell transplantation
E Allogeneic stem cell transplantation

Question 192

An asymptomatic 4-year-old girl presents with a groin mass. Physical examination shows a firm, matted, 3 × 5-cm mass in the left inguinal region. There is no other adenopathy or organomegaly. CT scans of the neck, chest, abdomen and pelvis show no other masses. A CBC and bilateral bone marrow aspirates are normal, as are the results of lumbar puncture. Biopsy of the mass shows a large cell lymphoma.

Q Which of the following would be optimal therapy for this patient?

A Nine weeks of CHOP (cyclophosphamide, doxorubicin, vincristine and prednisone) chemotherapy
B Nine weeks of CHOP plus intrathecal methotrexate
C Nine weeks of CHOP plus local irradiation
D Two years of multiagent chemotherapy
E Two years of multiagent chemotherapy plus intrathecal methotrexate

Question 193

A term, appropriate weight female is born after uncomplicated pregnancy and delivery. The mother is a vegetarian, is breast feeding her child and denies taking other medication during the pregnancy. She does not allow you to give the usual vitamin K 0.5 mg prior to discharge, despite your recommendations otherwise. At 2 months of age, the infant has 3 days of watery diarrhea. She presents 2 days later with an intracranial hemorrhage. Laboratory results show normal CBC and platelet count, but PT and APTT are both >100 s.

Q The most likely cause for this condition is:

A The mother was on anticonvulsants (dilantin) during pregnancy and did not tell you
B The mother is a vegetarian
C Undiagnosed cystic fibrosis
D Lack of vitamin K at birth and concurrent diarrheal illness

Question 194

A 12-month-old black infant is being evaluated for anemia. He has been healthy and his diet has been normal (consisting of iron-fortified formula and baby foods). The family history and physical examination are also normal. The hemoglobin is 10.4 g/dL, hematocrit 31%, reticulocyte count 1.3% and MCV 60 fL. Peripheral blood film shows microcytosis and occasional target cells. Hemoglobin electrophoresis shows 94% hemoglobin A, 4.5% hemoglobin F and 1.5% hemoglobin A_2.

Q Which of the following is the most likely diagnosis?

A Iron deficiency
B α Thalassemia trait
C β Thalassemia trait
D Anemia of inflammation
E The child is hematologically normal

Question 195

A 10-year-old girl presents with neck swelling and fevers for 1 month. She has lost 10 lb during that time. Physical examination shows bilateral cervical, axillary and inguinal adenopathy. Radiologic studies show a small anterior and middle mediastinal mass and enlarged para-aortic nodes. The liver and spleen appear normal. A CBC, bilateral bone marrow biopsies and liver function tests are normal. Her ESR is 86. Biopsy of a cervical node shows Hodgkin lymphoma, nodular sclerosing subtype.

Q Which of the following statements about the difference between Hodgkin lymphoma in children and adults is true?

A Children tolerate treatments less well than adults
B Children respond to treatments less well than adults
C Children respond to treatments better than adults
D Children are more likely to relapse than adults
E Children are more susceptible to complications of treatment because of incomplete growth and development

Question 196

A 6-year-old Spanish-American male with severe hemophilia B comes to the emergency room after falling two stories from an open window. He lost consciousness and has an obvious hematoma on the back of his head. While the nurse is arranging a stat CT scan, you are calculating his dose of recombinant factor IX. He weighs 20 kg. Recombinant factor IX calculation for dosing is higher than plasma-derived factor IX.

Q Which of the following is the appropriate dose of recombinant factor IX for this patient?

A 2500 U
B 3500 U
C 1250 U
D 1000 U

Question 197

A 3-year-old black girl with sickle cell anemia is evaluated for weakness and lethargy. For the past 2 days the child has also had a low-grade fever. Physical examination is normal except for pallor and a palpable spleen tip. Hemoglobin is 3.8 g/dL, hematocrit 10%, WBC count 8000/μL with 40% neutrophils and an otherwise normal differential, and platelet count 350,000/μL. Reticulocyte count is 0.3%.

Q Which of the following is the most likely diagnosis?

A Acute splenic sequestration crisis
B Vaso-occlusive crisis
C Aplastic crisis
D Megaloblastic crisis
E Hyperhemolytic crisis

Question 198

Q Which is the most likely side-effect of DDAVP administration in a 2-year-old male with type 1 von Willebrand disease (VWD) who will have PE tubes placed and an adenoidectomy performed for the indication of recurrent otitis media?

A Tachyphylaxis
B Thrombosis
C Hyponatremia and seizure
D Excessive urination

Question 199

A 2-year-old girl whose parents are both from Thailand is evaluated for fatigue and a CBC is performed. She has been healthy, takes vitamin supplementation and has a normal diet. Physical examination is normal. Her hemoglobin is 10.7 g/dL, hematocrit 31%, MCV 57 fL and reticulocyte count 0.8%. The WBC and platelet counts are normal. Peripheral blood smear shows a moderate number of target cells and some variation in red cell size and shape. A hemoglobin electrophoresis shows 74% hemoglobin A and 26% hemoglobin E.

Q Which of the following is the most likely diagnosis?

A Homozygous hemoglobin E disease
B Hemoglobin E β^o thalassemia
C Hemoglobin E β^+ thalassemia
D Hemoglobin E trait
E Hemoglobin E trait + α thalassemia trait

Question 200

A 29-year-old African-American man with hemoglobin SC undergoes laparoscopic cholecystectomy. The day after surgery he notices slight chest pain on deep inspiration. He subsequently complains of shortness of breath, bilateral pleuritic chest pain and inability to use his incentive spirometer effectively. On physical examination vital signs are: temperature 38.3°C, respiratory rate 28, pulse 118 and blood pressure 148/88 mmHg. On oxygen supplementation with $F\text{IO}_2$ of 40% the $P\text{O}_2$ is 60 mmHg. Chest examination reveals poor inspiratory effort and bilateral basilar crackles. There is no peripheral edema. The patient has not received any blood products in the perioperative period. The preoperative hemoglobin was 12.9 g/dL. The current hemoglobin is 11.2 g/dL, WBC 31,000/μL with 67% neutrophils, 13% bands, platelets 530,000/μL. Chest X-rays reveal diffuse patchy infiltrates. Broad-spectrum antibiotic therapy has been ordered.

Q Which of the following is the most appropriate next step in the management of this patient?

A Transfusion of packed red blood cells
B Administer D5 ½ normal saline (NS)
C Automated red blood cell exchange
D Phlebotomy of 1 unit of blood and then administration of 1 unit of packed red blood cells

Question 201

A 17-year-old Caucasian boy with hereditary spherocytosis seeks a second opinion about management of his disease. The patient has had multiple episodes of right upper quadrant pain and has been diagnosed with cholelithiasis by abdominal ultrasound. He complains of mild fatigue and has difficulty competing in high school sports. He experienced an episode of severe anemia at age 13 years, which was felt to represent an aplastic crisis. His only medication is folic acid 1 mg/day. Physical examination is remarkable for scleral icterus, a palpable spleen tip and mild jaundice. Laboratory data include Hb 8.8 g/dL, HCT 26% and reticulocyte count 9.8%. Review of the peripheral blood smear reveals a modest number of spherocytes. The total bilirubin is 2.9 mg/dL with a direct bilirubin of 0.4 mg/dL. Liver enzymes and liver synthetic function are otherwise normal. A repeat abdominal ultrasound reveals multiple gallstones, 1–3 mm in size, and mild splenomegaly.

Q Which of the following is the most appropriate management for this patient's condition:

A Splenectomy
B Cholecystectomy
C Combined splenectomy and cholecystectomy
D Increase the dosage of folic acid to 5 mg/day

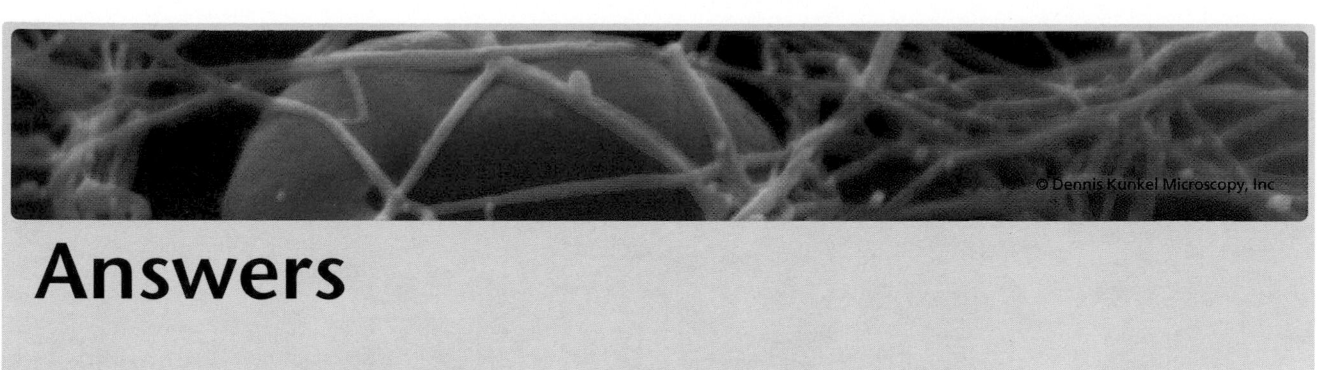

Answers

Answer to question 1: D

Educational objective

To recognize the most sensitive test for diagnosing chronic myeloid leukemia in lymphoid blast crisis

Critique

The Philadelphia chromosome, a balanced translocation involving the *BCR* gene on chromosome 22 and the *ABL* gene on chromosome 9, is the defining chromosomal abnormality in chronic myeloid leukemia (CML). This translocation is also present in approximately half of cases of acute lymphoblastic leukemia (ALL) in adults. Molecular characterization of the fusion transcript that is created by the translocation has demonstrated heterogeneity in the exact site of the translocation breakpoints. Patients with CML usually harbor a translocation that encodes a protein with a molecular weight of 210 kDa. The fusion transcript present in patients with *de novo* ALL usually encodes a protein with a molecular weight of 190 kDa. Patients with CML may progress to lymphoid blast crisis at variable latency. The t(9;22) in these cases of ALL usually encodes the p210. Using molecular techniques, CML in lymphoid blast crisis and *de novo* Philadelphia-positive ALL can be distinguished. This is accomplished by performing RT-PCR on the leukemic cells using primers that are specific for the different translocations. These primers are designed for application to RT-PCR. The primers span large introns that are too far apart for PCR amplification of the relevant region in genomic DNA. While in theory Western blot analysis could be used to distinguish p190 and p210, PCR-based studies are simpler and more practical to perform and interpret.

References

Jones CD, Yeung C, Zehnder JL. Comprehensive validation of a real-time quantitative *bcr-abl* assay for clinical laboratory use. Am J Clin Pathol. 2003;120:42–8.

Pane F, Intrieri M, Quintarelli C, Izzo B, Muccioli GC, Salvatore F. BCR/ABL genes and leukemic phenotype: from molecular mechanisms to clinical correlations. Oncogene. 2002;21:8652–67.

Answer to question 2: C

Educational objective

To diagnose hypoplastic myelodysplastic syndrome on the basis of morphology

Critique

The distinction between aplastic anemia (AA) and hypoplastic myelodysplastic syndrome (MDS) is difficult. Although these two disorders probably constitute distinct diseases with differing rates of evolution to acute leukemia, there is increasing evidence that suggests that immunologic mechanisms similar to those operative in AA may contribute to the cytopenias of both hypo- and hypercellular MDS (even in the absence of preceding AA). In addition to dysplasias typical of MDS, such as the Pelger–Huet abnormality of blood neutrophils and dysplastic megakaryocytes, ALIPs are indicative of a hypoplastic MDS. In a normal bone marrow biopsy, myeloid precursors are proximal to the trabecular region, and erythroid and megakaryocytic precursors tend to be intertrabecular. This cell distribution may be reversed in patients with MDS. Sometimes the only way to distinguish between these two disorders is by detection of an abnormal karyotype. If hypoplastic MDS is diagnosed, stem cell transplant would be the only curative option. However, immunosuppressive therapy can produce responses in patients with both hypo- and hypercellular MDS and the diagnosis of hypocellular MDS does not preclude treatment with antithymocyte globulin or cyclosporine. Vitamin B_{12} or folate deficiency can cause pancytopenia and macrocytosis. Vitamin B_{12} or folate deficiency is a consideration in the patient with pancytopenia and macrocytosis (and levels should be checked in patients such as the one described here). Nonetheless, the absence of macrocytosis in this patient with significant cytopenia and the bone marrow appearance suggest that vitamin B_{12} deficiency is not the most likely diagnosis; megaloblastic marrow morphology and subtle dysplasia can be seen with vitamin B_{12} deficiency.

References

Barrett J, Sauntharajah Y, Molldrem J. Myelodysplastic syndrome and aplastic anemia: distinct entities of diseases linked by a common pathophysiology. Semin Hematol. 2000;37:15–29.

Saunthararajah Y, Nakamura R, Nam J, Robyn J, Loberiza F, Maciejewski JP, et al. HLA DR15 is over-represented in myelodysplastic syndrome and aplastic anemia, and predicts a response to immunosuppression in myelodysplastic syndrome. Blood. 2002;100:1570–4.

Answer to question 3: (a) D, (b) B

Educational objective

To recognize the cause of and manage thrombocytopenia in a patient with HIV

Critique

This patient has a normal WBC, mild anemia and significant thrombocytopenia. This makes it unlikely that the thrombocytopenia is caused by HIV-induced marrow failure (in which pancytopenia would be found), and more likely that the thrombocytopenia is caused by peripheral destruction of platelets. Idiopathic thrombocytopenic purpura (ITP) is very common in patients with HIV. Thrombotic thrombocytopenic purpura (TTP) usually presents with more severe anemia, in addition to fever, neurologic abnormalities and renal insufficiency. Vitamin B_{12} deficiency more commonly presents with macrocytic anemia.

Initiation of highly active antiretroviral therapy is an effective way to increase the platelet count in patients with HIV-associated ITP. The platelet count usually improves within 1–2 months. Oprelvekin (IL-11) is indicated for chemotherapy-induced thrombocytopenia, but would not be indicated in ITP. Transfused platelets have a short survival in ITP, and would not be indicated in this nonbleeding patient. As other therapeutic interventions are often successful for HIV-associated ITP, the option of splenectomy would be reserved for later in this patient's clinical course.

Reference

Scaradavou A. HIV-related thrombocytopenia. Blood Rev. 2002;16:73–6.

Answer to question 4: E

Educational objective

To recognize zinc excess as a cause of microcytic anemia

Critique

Excess dietary zinc can lead to copper deficiency by decreasing copper absorption. Copper is part of two metalloproteins, ceruloplasmin and hephestin, both of which maintain iron in its Fe^{3+} state such that it can be bound to transferrin and subsequently used for erythropoiesis. Copper deficiency leads to a microcytic anemia that does not respond to supplemental iron. Ginseng, turmeric and echinacea do not affect erythropoiesis. Ascorbic acid can facilitate dietary iron absorption.

Reference

Ramadurai J, Shapiro C, Kozloff M, Telfer M. Zinc abuse and sideroblastic anemia. Am J Hematol. 1993;42:227–8.

Answer to question 5: A

Educational objective

To recognize *Helicobacter pylori* as an important cause of iron deficiency anemia in children refractory to supplemental iron

Critique

Helicobacter pylori infection is known to affect both iron and ferritin levels, which are reduced in both adults and children infected with this organism. This seems to occur independently of active gastrointestinal bleeding. The mechanism for this association is not well understood although microbiological studies suggest that the *H. pylori*-infected antrum acts as a sequestering focus for serum iron by means of outer membrane receptors of the bacterium, which *in vitro* are able to capture and utilize iron from human lactoferrin for growth. In one study of children, 14% of children infected with *H. pylori* were iron deficient as compared with 3% of unaffected children. Treating *H. pylori* in these individuals leads to an appropriate response to oral iron therapy. Cobalamin or folate will not resolve iron deficiency anemia. Ferrous sulfate, ferrous fumarate and ferrous gluconate all appear to be equally effective hematinic agents.

References

Kostaki M, Fessatou S, Karpathios T. Refractory iron-deficiency anemia due to silent *Helicobacter pylori* gastritis in children. Eur J Pediatr. 2003;162:177–9.

Sugiyama T, Tsuchida M, Yokata K, Shimodan M, Asaka M. Improvement of long-standing iron-deficiency anemia in adults after eradication of *Helicobacter pylori* infection. Intern Med. 2002;41:491–4.

Answer to question 6: D

Educational objective

To recognize spur cell anemia as a cause of hemolysis in end-stage liver disease and identify proper treatment

Critique

This patient has late-stage alcoholic liver disease and the presence of an acquired hemolytic anemia. In severe liver disease, altered cholesterol metabolism leads to acanthocyte formation and subsequent hemolysis. Unfortunately, the only definitive treatment to reverse this condition is liver transplantation. Erythropoietin might be helpful, but the reticulocyte count is already elevated and it will likely not provide adequate compensation for the hemolytic process.

Prednisone and rituximab are useful in autoimmune hemolytic anemia but would not improve spur cell anemia. Plasmapheresis has been used in cold agglutinin disease with hemodynamic compromise but would not be effective in this clinical setting. In addition, when plasmapheresis is performed in liver disease (correcting a coagulopathy as a bridge to transplantation), fresh frozen plasma would be a better replacement product, given the likely underlying coagulopathy associated with end-stage liver disease.

References

Chitale AA, Sterling RK, Post AB, Silver BJ, Mulligan DC, Schulak JA. Resolution of spur cell anemia with liver transplantation: a case report and review of the literature. Transplantation. 1998;65:993–5.

Doll DC, Doll NJ. Spur cell anemia. South Med J. 1982;75:1205–10.

Melrose WD, Bell PA, Jupe DM, Baikie MJ. Alcohol-associated haemolysis in Zieve's syndrome: a clinical and laboratory study of five cases. Clin Lab Haematol. 1990;12:159–67.

Answer to question 7: C

Educational objective

To recognize medications that can affect the neutrophil count

Critique

Lithium, a monovalent cation, induces neutrophilia in at least 20% of patients who receive standard doses for manic-depressive illness. The exact mechanism is unknown; however, the effect is independent of the plasma drug level and dosage adjustment is not required in the absence of other adverse effects. Imipramine, a tricyclic antidepressant, and clozapine, a tricyclic dibenzodiazepine derivative atypical antipsychotic agent, are potential causes of neutropenia but not neutrophilia. Because some patients receiving clozapine have developed agranulocytosis, routine monitoring of the neutrophil count is recommended. Chronic myeloid leukemia (CML) is unlikely in this case in the absence of circulating immature myeloid cells, basophilia, thrombocytosis and splenomegaly. However, CML would be a consideration if the patient is not taking lithium and has persistent unexplained neutrophilia. Alcohol ingestion does not induce leukocytosis. Rather, chronic alcohol abuse can lead to neutropenia because of hypersplenism (secondary to liver disease and portal hypertension) or folate deficiency.

References

Boggs DR, Joyce RA. The hematopoietic effects of lithium. Semin Hematol. 1983;20:129–38.

Reding MT, Hibbs JR, Morrison VA, Swaim WR, Filice GA. Diagnosis and outcome of 100 consecutive patients with extreme granulocytic leukocytosis. Am J Med. 1998;104:12–6.

van der Klauw MM, Goudsmit R, Halie MR, van't Veer MB, Herings RM, Wilson JH, et al. A population-based case–cohort study of drug-associated agranulocytosis. Arch Intern Med. 1999;159:369–74.

Answer to question 8: B

Educational objective

To recognize the pathophysiologic mechanism of MDS

Critique

The classic bone marrow finding in MDS is hypercellularity, in contrast to the marked cytopenias seen in the peripheral blood. This fits well with the pathophysiology of these disorders, which can be best characterized as ineffective hematopoiesis rather than a lack of hematopoietic activity. Patients who have received previous chemotherapy, especially alkylating agents, are at higher risk for the development of MDS. The latency period is typically 5–10 years, in contrast to therapy-related acute myeloid leukemia (AML) resulting from topoisomerase II inhibitors, which has a much shorter latency period. Cytogenetic studies are extremely important in MDS to determine prognosis, and have been incorporated into the International Prognostic Scoring System (IPSS) for this reason.

References

Greenberg P, Cox C, LeBeau MM, Fenaux P, Morel P, Sanz G et al. International scoring system for evaluating prognosis in myelodysplastic syndromes. Blood. 1997;89:2079–88.

Heaney ML, Golde DW. Myelodysplasia. N Engl J Med. 1999;340:1649–60.

Answer to question 9: E

Educational objective

To recognize the optimal induction chemotherapy for younger adults with AML

Critique

Since the late 1960s, a series of studies have been conducted that have established an induction regimen which can be considered as standard for those patients not participating in a clinical trial. Daunorubicin in a regimen of 45–60 mg/m^2/day for 3 days, given together with cytarabine 100 mg/m^2/day for 7 days by continuous infusion, is commonly used. In younger adults, a 45-mg/m^2 dose has been shown to be superior to a 30-mg/m^2 dose. 90 mg/m^2/day for 3 days has been studied, but has not been compared with lower doses and cannot be considered the standard of care. Regarding the doses of cytarabine, 200 mg/m^2 has been compared with 100 mg/m^2 and they appear equivalent. No studies have suggested that higher doses of cytarabine in induction are clearly beneficial.

References

Rai KR, Holland JF, Glidewell OJ, et al. Treatment of acute myelocytic leukemia: a study by Cancer and Leukemia Group B. Blood. 1981;58:1203–12.

Rowe JM, Tallman MS. Intensifying induction therapy in acute myeloid leukemia: has a new standard of care emerged? Blood. 1997;90:2121–6.

Yates J, Glidewell O, Wiernik P, et al. Cytosine arabinoside with daunorubicin or Adriamycin for therapy of acute myelocytic leukemia: a CALGB study. Blood. 1982;60:454–62.

Answer to question 10: C

Educational objective

To recognize the characteristic chromosomal abnormality in childhood ALL

Critique

Between 60 and 70% of infants with ALL have a translocation involving the 11q23 region. The partner chromosome varies but a t(4;11) is the most frequent finding. These individuals have more frequent and more pronounced hepatosplenomegaly and adenopathy, higher WBC and an increased risk of CNS disease when compared with older children with ALL. The blasts are usually CD10$^-$ (CALLA; common ALL antigen). Event-free survival is poor regardless of the partner chromosome. Infants >9 months at diagnosis of ALL have physical findings, laboratory findings and prognosis more akin to those of typical childhood ALL. The translocations t(1;19), t(9;22) and hypodiploidy are rare in infants with ALL.

References

Pui C-H, Gaynon PS, Boyett JM, Chessells JM, Baruchel A, Kamps W, et al. Outcome of treatment in childhood acute lymphoblastic leukaemia with rearrangements of the 11q23 region. Lancet. 2002;359:1909–15.

Reaman GH, Sposto R, Sensel MG, Lange BJ, Feusner JH, Heerema NA, et al. Treatment outcome and prognostic factors for infants with acute lymphoblastic leukemia treated on two consecutive trials of the Children's Cancer Group. J Clin Oncol. 1999;17:1–11.

Answer to question 11: A

Educational objective

To understand the phenotypic and molecular markers of disease progression and prognosis in CLL

Critique

Prognosis in CLL can be estimated by disease stage, phenotype and molecular characteristics. Early stage (Rai stage 0, Binet stage A) patients, such as the individual in this case, have median survivals of >10 years. Pre- and postgerminal center CLL subtypes are recognized, the former usually expressing CD38 and ZAP-70 and associated with a shorter time to progression and survival than the postgerminal center subtype (CD38$^-$, ZAP-70$^-$). Several molecular markers, best identified by FISH analysis, are also predictive of disease prognosis. Isolated 13q deletions have an excellent prognosis, with median survivals beyond 8–10 years. This patient has uniformly favorable clinical features and is unlikely to require therapy for 5 or more years. None of these markers reliably predicts large cell lymphoma or prolymphocytic leukemia transformation.

References

Crespo M, Bosch BS, Villamar N, Bellosillo B, Colomer D, Rozman M, et al. ZAP-70 expression as a surrogate for immunoglobulin variable region mutations in chronic lymphocytic leukemia. N Engl J Med. 2003;348:1764–75.

Dohner H, Stilgenbauer S, Benner A, Leupolt E, Krober A, Bullinger L, et al. Genomic aberrations and survival in chronic lymphocytic leukemia. N Engl J Med. 2000;343:1910–6.

Answer to question 12: B

Educational objective

To recognize that a one antigen-mismatched related donor is preferable to an HLA-identical unrelated donor

Critique

The patient and her sister share five of six HLA A, B and C antigens and are matched at class II level. Although they are mismatched on one locus, related donor transplants with one antigen mismatch have outcomes similar to fully matched sibling transplants. Thus, this donor would be preferred over an unrelated HLA-identical donor and over a one antigen-matched sibling. Although autologous transplantation could be considered, it does not have the same potential for long-term disease-free survival that allogeneic transplantation does in this clinical situation.

Reference

Beatty PG, Clift RA, Mickelson EM, Nisperos BB, Flournoy N, Martin PJ, et al. Marrow transplantation from related donors other than HLA-identical siblings. N Engl J Med. 1985;313:765–71.

Answer to question 13: E

Educational objective

To manage chronic thrombocytopenia in a patient with ITP

Critique

The objective of this question is to emphasize that the goal of treatment for ITP is to prevent bleeding, not to cure the illness. This principle is the foundation for the practice of observation, without drug treatment, for asymptomatic patients with only moderate thrombocytopenia. However, in patients with severe and symptomatic thrombocytopenia, aggressive treatment to alter the course of the disease is necessary.

In this patient, the diagnosis of ITP is assumed to be accurate, and the course is typical for ITP in adults. Initial treatment, at the time of diagnosis, was appropriate because of the severity of the thrombocytopenia. Splenectomy was the appropriate second-line treatment when initial prednisone was not associated with a sustained remission. Initial response to splenectomy is complete in most patients, approximately 70%, and apparently sustained in most patients who initially respond.

Treatment modalities for ITP other than prednisone and splenectomy have a poor record of success and none has been studied in randomized controlled clinical trials. Therefore it is unknown if the benefits of these treatments exceed the risks. Even with rituximab, currently the most popular treatment for patients with refractory ITP, no response is more frequent than remission. Persistence or development of an accessory spleen has been reported to cause recurrent thrombocytopenia, but reports of responses following accessory splenectomy are very rare, suggesting that responses may be coincidental. If this patient had a platelet count <10,000/μL and evidence of bleeding, then further treatment with immunosuppressive agents would be appropriate. However, in an asymptomatic patient with moderate thrombocytopenia, there is no indication for treatment. It is a common experience among patients with chronic persistent thrombocytopenia resulting from ITP that complications of treatment exceed their problems from bleeding. The most cautious and appropriate management for this patient is to taper and discontinue her prednisone and observe her. Further treatment is not necessary unless she has clinically important bleeding symptoms, or perhaps for very severe thrombocytopenia, i.e. a platelet count <10,000/μL.

References

George JN, Kojouri K, Perdue JJ, Vesely SK. Management of chronic refractory idiopathic thrombocytopenic purpura. Semin Hematol. 2000;37:290–8.

Provan D, Newland A. Fifty years of idiopathic thrombocytopenic purpura (ITP): management of refractory ITP in adults. Br J Haematol. 2002;118:933–44.

Vesely SK, Perdue JJ, Rizvi MA, Terrell DR, George JN. Management of adult patients with idiopathic thrombocytopenic purpura after failure of splenectomy. A systematic review. Ann Intern Med. 2004;140:112–20.

Answer to question 14: C

Educational objective

To recognize the presentation of a delayed hemolytic transfusion reaction

Critique

This is an example of a delayed hemolytic transfusion reaction (DHTR). The patient had formed an alloantibody (in the actual case in this question it was an antibody against Jk^a, one of the Kidd system antigens) after exposure to red cells during his previous surgery 20 years before. This patient's alloantibody had decayed to subdetectable levels over time, as is common for Kidd antibodies, and so was not found during pretransfusion antibody screening. After exposure to the Jk^a donor units (in this case 9 of the 12 units were Jk^a positive), the alloantibody re-emerged during an anamnestic response, causing an extravascular hemolytic reaction. When primary alloantibody formation is induced, the appearance of detectable levels of the offending IgG antibody is seen in a few weeks, and most of the transfused cells have been cleared by then through senescence. The emergence of an alloantibody that does not cause hemolysis is termed a delayed serologic transfusion reaction. Sometimes the alloantibody can be detected by retesting the pretransfusion sample using more sensitive methods that are not commonly employed in routine antibody screening, but the best way to detect DHTR antibodies is by testing a post-transfusion sample for the new (re-emerging) alloantibody. Although ABO mistakes causing hemolytic transfusion reactions do happen, chiefly through mislabeled samples or inattention to proper patient identification, these reactions cause immediate symptoms and would not be under consideration here. If there had been other clinical signs and symptoms that could have explained the jaundice and dropping hemoglobin, such as bleeding or infection, the recognition that this was a DHTR could have been delayed or missed. This is one reason why antibody screens are required after a transfusion, so as not to miss new alloantibodies.

References

Ness PM, Shirey RS, Weinstein MH, King KE. An animal model for delayed hemolytic transfusion reactions. Transfus Med Rev. 2001;15:305–17.

Pineda AA, Vamvakas EC, Gorden LD, Winters JL, Moore SB. Trends in the incidence of delayed hemolytic and delayed serologic transfusion reactions. Transfusion. 1999;39:1097–103.

Shulman IA, Downes KA, Sazama K, Maffei LM. Pretransfusion compatibility testing for red blood cell administration. Curr Opin Hematol. 2001;8:397–404.

Answer to question 15: E

Educational objective

To evaluate a patient with a prolonged prothrombin time and prolonged activated partial thromboplastin time

Critique

The most common cause of a prolonged APTT that does not correct in a mixing study is a lupus anticoagulant, and this assay should be completed. In patients with lupus anticoagulants, an associated prolonged prothrombin time that does correct in the 1 : 1 mixing is most likely caused by a second antibody directed against prothrombin (factor II) rather than decreased synthesis or a congenital deficiency. This antibody (separate from the lupus anticoagulant) binds to an area of the prothrombin molecule that does not inhibit the active site (thus the mixing study does not indicate an inhibitor), and the decrease in prothrombin is caused by clearance of prothrombin as part of the immune complex. A lupus anticoagulant alone would not account for this much prolongation of the prothrombin time. Low factor VIII or an inhibitor to factor VIII would also not account for the prolonged prothrombin time. Although deficiencies of factors V, X and II would give a prolongation of both the prothrombin time and APTT, correction of both tests in mixing studies would be expected.

References

Fleck RA, Rapaport SI, Rao VM. Antiprothrombin antibodies and the lupus anticoagulant. Blood. 1988;72:512–9.

Pernod G, Arvieux J, Carpentier PH, Pascal M, Bosson J, Luc Benoît P. Successful treatment of lupus anticoagulant hypoprothrombinemia syndrome using intravenous immunoglobulins. Thromb Haemost. 1997;78:969–70.

Answer to question 16: A

Educational objective

To recognize the importance of effective communication with a referring physician in consultation

Critique

People commonly seek a second opinion for hematologic disorders. The consultant giving a second opinion should review the primary data and confirm the history and physical examination. A telephone call to the primary hematologist toward the end of the interview will help to verify the accuracy of the received information and permit a two-way exchange regarding the second hematologist's recommendations. A videotape of the encounter might help the patient avoid misunderstanding, but it does not ensure clear two-way communication between the referring physician and the first hematologist. Similarly, a follow-up call to the patient may not improve communication to the first hematologist. Currently, there are no firm guidelines for communication of HIPPA protected information by nonencrypted e-mail.

Reference

Kitchens CS. The consultative process. In: Kitchens CS, Alving BM, Kessler CM, eds. Consultative Hemostasis and Thrombosis. Philadelphia, PA: W.B. Saunders, 2002.

Answer to question 17: A

Educational objective

To recognize the most sensitive test for detecting relapse in CML

Critique

The most sensitive way to detect residual leukemia cells in a patient with the t(9;22) is to perform RT-PCR for the *BCR-ABL* translocation. RT-PCR can reliably detect as few as 1 in 10^4 cells. Several studies have established that RT-PCR performed on peripheral blood is as reliable as studies of bone marrow, obviating the need for repeated bone marrow aspirations. Conventional cytogenetics and FISH can be used, but they are less sensitive. Cytogenetics will detect the Philadelphia chromosome, but because the laboratory rarely counts more than 100 cells, it only detects relapse at the 1% level. FISH for the *BCR-ABL* translocation is more sensitive than cytogenetics. Its sensitivity is again dependent on the number of cells that are counted, but it is rarely useful in detecting disease at a level of less than 1 cell in 10^3. Flow cytometry is not a useful study in CML and is less sensitive than RT-PCR in detecting the presence of residual acute leukemia cells.

References

Eder M, Battmer K, Kafert S, Stucki A, Ganser A, Hertenstein B. Monitoring of BCR-ABL expression using real-time RT-PCR in CML after bone marrow or peripheral blood stem cell transplantation. Leukemia. 1999;13:1383–9.

Lee M, Khouri I, Champlin R, et al. Detection of minimal residual disease by polymerase chain reaction of *bcr-abl* transcripts in chronic myelogenous leukemia following allogeneic bone marrow transplantation. Br J Hematol. 1992;82:708.

Answer to question 18: E

Educational objective

To recognize the causes of erythrocytosis

Critique

Polycythemia vera (PV) is a myeloproliferative disorder characterized by a high red cell mass due to autonomous erythroid overproduction. PV is commonly associated with a low or undetectable serum erythropoietin (Epo) level, elevated platelet count and palpable splenomegaly. Other diagnostic features of PV include: absence of causes for secondary polycythemia, leukocytosis, endogenous erythroid colony growth of peripheral blood progenitors and a clonal karyotypic abnormality on marrow cytogenetics. In this case, the hemoglobin level of >18.5 g/dL indicates true polycythemia, as this high value could not be achieved by plasma volume contraction alone. Thus, a formal red cell mass study would not be useful or indicated. An elevated red cell mass rules out Gaisböck syndrome, which refers to relative erythrocytosis due to decreased plasma volume, often in patients with hypertension. Secondary polycythemias must be considered; however, in contrast to this case, these are usually associated with elevated Epo levels. Secondary polycythemias are most commonly caused by hypoxemia, which, in turn, stimulates increased Epo production. Systemic hypoxemia may be caused by chronic lung disease, residing at high altitude, cyanotic congenital heart disease, chronic carbon monoxide exposure (from heavy long-term smoking or working in a poorly ventilated automobile garage) or chronic hypoventilation (from morbid obesity or sleep apnea). Local renal hypoxemia, caused by renal cysts, tumour or renal artery stenosis, may also cause elevated Epo and secondary polycythemia. Chuvash-type polycythemia, originally described in individuals from the Russian Chuvash population, is caused by a mutation in the von Hippel–Lindau (*VHL*) gene leading to defective oxygen sensing and secondary Epo overproduction.

Reference

Tefferi A. Polycythemia vera: a comprehensive review and clinical recommendations. Mayo Clin Proc. 2003;78:174–94.

Answer to question 19: A

Educational objective

To identify Fanconi anemia as the cause of aplastic anemia

Critique

Approximately 30% of patients with Fanconi anemia lack typical physical findings, and approximately 10% of patients present at ages older than 16 years. Therefore, it is reasonable to consider Fanconi anemia as a cause of aplastic anemia in young adult patients. In patients without the classic constellation of musculoskeletal or dermatological features, the diagnosis relies on chromosome breakage analysis in which phytohemagglutinin-stimulated peripheral blood lymphocytes are cultured with and without clastogenic agents (DEB or mitomycin C). Patients with Fanconi anemia have an increased frequency of chromosome abnormalities when exposed to clastogenic agents. The percentage of cells in G2M arrest as assessed by flow cytometry is an alternative endpoint in these analyses of DEB-treated cells—patients with Fanconi anemia will have an increased percentage of cells in G2M arrest. A myeloperoxidase stain can be used to help distinguish between myeloblasts versus lymphoblasts if an increased percentage of blasts is noted on a Giemsa-stained marrow aspirate smear.

Reference

Venkitaraman AR. A growing network of cancer-susceptibility genes. N Engl J Med. 2003;348:1917–9.

Answer to question 20: C

Educational objective

To begin acute therapy for severe anemia in a patient with myelodysplasia

Critique

This patient has angina, likely exacerbated by his severe anemia. Transfusion of 2 IU of PRBC will promptly increase his HCT. Patients with myelodysplasia have an approximately 20% chance of responding to an erythroid growth factor with a 1–2 g/dL increase in the hemoglobin, but response is usually seen during the second month of therapy. The use of an erythroid growth factor plus filgrastim increases the chance of response to approximately 40%, but again the time frame is within 4–8 weeks. Prednisone would not be appropriate therapy for this patient.

Reference

Kasper C, Zahner J, Sayer HG. Recombinant human erythropoietin in combined treatment with granulocyte- or granulocyte-macrophage colony-stimulating factor in patients with myelodysplastic syndromes. J Cancer Res Clin Oncol. 2002;128:499–502.

Answer to question 21: D

Educational objective

To calculate iron replacement requirements for a target hemoglobin concentration

Critique

To calculate replacement doses of iron, it is important to remember that 1 mL of blood contains approximately 1 mg of iron. Further, the total blood volume is 65 mL/kg and hemoglobin (Hb) contains approximately 0.34% iron by weight. Therefore:

$$\text{Iron deficit (g)} = (\text{target Hb} - \text{actual Hb [g/dL]})/100 \times \text{weight (kg)} \times 65 \times 0.0034$$

$$\text{Iron deficit (mg)} = (\text{target Hb} - \text{actual Hb}) \times \text{weight (kg)} \times 2.2$$

$$\text{Iron deficit (mg)} = (\text{target Hb} - \text{actual Hb}) \times \text{weight (lb)}$$

This represents the amount of iron needed to make up the extra red blood cell (RBC) mass. To this amount, storage iron must be added, which is approximately 600 mg for women and 1000 mg for men. For this patient, this represents 750 [(12 – 7) × 150] mg of iron to replenish Hb in addition to 600 mg of storage iron for a total amount of 1350 mg. It should be remembered that only approximately 5–10% of oral iron is actually absorbed, so oral replacement would require a much greater amount of elemental iron.

References

Fairbanks VF, Beutler E. Iron deficiency. In: Beutler E, Lichtman MA, Coller B, Kipps TJ, Seligsohn U, eds. William's Hematology, 6th edn. McGraw-Hill, 2001.

Wallerstein RO. Intravenous iron-dextran complex. Blood. 1968;32:690–5.

Answer to question 22: B

Educational objective

To treat the anemia associated with congenital dyserythropoietic anemia

Critique

The congenital dyserythropoietic anemias (CDAs) are characterized by anemia, jaundice, multinucleated erythroblasts in the marrow and iron overload. The disease usually presents by age 6 years, with more than half of patients having severe anemia and jaundice. Iron overload is common and occurs independently of hemochromatosis genotype. Hemolysis occurs secondary to ineffective erythropoiesis and is not related to complement. Splenectomy has been shown to be effective in ameliorating anemia and jaundice in these patients. Recently, it has been shown that some patients with type II CDA may have defects in cellular glycosylation. Although these patients may require iron chelation to control their iron overload, chelation does not improve anemia in this disorder.

References

Iolascon A, Delaunay J, Wickramasinghe SN, Perrotta S, Gigante M, Camaschella C. Natural history of congenital dyserythropoietic anemia type II. Blood. 2001;98:1258–60.

Marks PW, Mitus AJ. Congenital dyserythropoietic anemias. Am J Hematol. 1996;51:55–63.

Answer to question 23: C

Educational objective

To recognize the acute clinical presentation and treatment of acquired methemoglobinemia

Critique

This young child develops cyanosis, normal oxygen tension, decreased oxygen saturation and chocolate-appearing blood soon after the administration of benzocaine spray. This constellation of findings strongly suggests methemoglobinemia. Confirmation laboratory testing is recommended, although treatment should not be delayed. This condition is treated with methylene blue, which serves as an electron carrier and reverses the cyanosis. Methylene blue should be avoided in patients with known glucose-6-phosphate dehydrogenase (G6PD) deficiency, as it can accelerate hemolysis. Treatment is necessary as this patient is symptomatic and peripheral oxygenation is compromised. Red blood cell exchange and methylprednisolone would be ineffective therapy for acquired methemoglobinemia.

Hyberbaric oxygen could be considered if the patient did not respond or deteriorated after treatment with methylene blue, the initial treatment of choice.

References

Aepfelbacher FC, Breen P, Manning WJ. Methemoglobinemia and topical pharyngeal anesthesia. N Engl J Med. 2003;348:85–6.

Groeper K, Katcher K, Tobias JD. Anesthetic management of a patient with methemoglobinemia. South Med J. 2003;96:504–9.

Wright RO, Lewander WJ, Woolf AD. Methemoglobinemia: etiology, pharmacology, and clinical management. Ann Emerg Med. 1999;34:646–56.

Answer to question 24: B

Educational objective

To treat polycythemia vera in a pregnant woman with a history of thrombosis

Critique

Standard therapy for a woman with PV includes phlebotomy to maintain the hematocrit <42%, or <37% if in the third trimester of pregnancy. In addition, daily low-dose aspirin, at 100 mg/day, is recommended for thromboprophylaxis in patients without contraindications or bleeding risk. Low-dose aspirin (81–250 mg/day) will also likely benefit this patient's symptoms and signs of erythromelalgia (in her fingers and toes). The additional major consideration for adjunctive therapy in this patient relates to her risk of pregnancy-associated thrombotic complications. Cytoreductive therapy, to normalize the platelet count, should be considered if she has previously suffered a thrombotic event or adverse pregnancy outcome with an elevated platelet count (e.g. >600,000/μL). If indicated, interferon-α is the platelet-lowering agent of choice during pregnancy because it is effective and safe. Hydroxyurea and anagrelide are potentially teratogenic and are therefore contraindicated during pregnancy. In this case, the platelet count is not significantly elevated and cytoreductive therapy is, therefore, not indicated. However, her previous history of thrombosis imparts an increased risk of arterial or venous thromboemboli (hazard ratio of approximately 5) related to PV, independent of the added risk of pregnancy. Thus, to minimize this risk, prophylactic heparin, usually given as low-molecular-weight heparin, should be started and continued through 6 weeks' postpartum.

References

Delage R, Demers C, Cantin G, Roy J. Treatment of essential thrombocythemia during pregnancy with interferon-α. Obstet Gynecol. 1996;87(Part2):814–7.

Griesshammer M, Bergmann L, Pearson T. Fertility, pregnancy and the management of myeloproliferative disorders. Bailliere's Clin Haematol. 1998;11:859–74.

Spivak JL, Barosi G, Tognoni G, Barbui T, Finazzi G, Marchioli R, et al. Chronic Myeloproliferative Disorders. Hematology (Am Soc Hematol Educ Program), 2003:200–24.

Answer to question 25: A

Educational objective

To diagnose large granular lymphocyte leukemia

Critique

Severe neutropenia (<500/μL) associated with lymphocytosis in a patient with palpable splenomegaly and a history of rheumatoid arthritis is highly suggestive of either large granular lymphocyte (LGL) leukemia or Felty syndrome. LGL leukemia is most commonly associated with clonal expansion of $CD3^+$ T lymphocytes and less commonly (10–20% of cases) associated with clonal $CD3^-$, $CD56^+$ natural killer (NK) cells. Felty syndrome, which consists of splenomegaly, neutropenia and rheumatoid arthritis (usually with high-titer rheumatoid factor), may, in a minority of patients, be associated with increased numbers of reactive (nonclonal) $CD3^+$ LGLs. Neutropenia with LGL leukemia appears to be related to Fas-mediated neutrophil cell death, whereas neutropenia with Felty syndrome is predominantly caused by autoimmune destruction secondary to various antineutrophil antibodies. In the peripheral blood smear, LGLs appear as atypical lymphocytes with prominent azurophilic cytoplasmic granules. They are identified as either T or NK cells by immunophenotypic analyses. However, the T-cell receptor gene rearrangement study is required to discriminate clonal $CD3^+$ LGLs from a reactive polyclonal population. Cytogenetic abnormalities are not commonly found with LGL leukemia. Marrow morphology typically reveals a maturation arrest in the myeloid series and variable infiltration with atypical lymphocytes or LGLs; however, these changes are not specific for LGL leukemia and could reflect reactive lymphocytosis with autoimmune or drug-induced neutropenia. Immunophenotypic studies and B-cell clonality assays would be helpful in diagnosing a B-cell lymphoproliferative disorder, such as hairy cell leukemia (HCL), chronic lymphocytic leukemia (CLL) or peripheralized non-Hodgkin lymphoma (NHL). HCL more commonly presents with pancytopenia, and with low numbers of circulating hairy cells. Similarly, peripheralized NHL or CLL are not usually associated with isolated severe neutropenia.

References

Lamy T, Loughran TP Jr. Clinical features of large granular lymphocyte leukemia. Semin Hematol. 2003;40:185–95.

Starkebaum G. Chronic neutropenia associated with autoimmune disease. Semin Hematol. 2002;39:121–7.

Answer to question 26: B

Educational objective

To recognize the high risk of perioperative thrombotia complications in patients with polycythemia vera and poorly controlled blood counts

Critique

This patient has many features suggestive of polycythemia vera (PV), including a high red cell mass (indicated by the preoperative hemoglobin >18.5 g/dL), palpable splenomegaly, thrombocytosis and consistent peripheral blood morphologic abnormalities (i.e. basophilia and giant platelets). Poorly controlled PV, with the high hematocrit and platelet count, at the time of major surgery imparts an 80% risk of postoperative bleeding and thrombotic complications. By comparison, patients with PV whose counts are normalized many weeks before surgery have only modestly increased risk. The pathogenesis of arterial and venous thromboemboli with PV is multifactorial, and relates to hyperviscosity secondary to erythrocytosis, dysfunctional platelets and hemostatic effects of activated granulocytes. The arterial event suffered by this patient is not likely due to a factor V Leiden mutation, surgery-induced hypercoagulability or stasis with postoperative immobilization because those conditions predispose to venous thromboemboli. The high postoperative platelet count in this case argues against disseminated intravascular coagulopathy (DIC) as a mechanism. Treatment of this patient should include therapeutic infusion of standard heparin, phlebotomy to normalize the hematocrit, and consideration of plateletpheresis to normalize the platelet count and minimize the chance of further thromboembolic complications.

Reference

Spivak JL. Polycythemia vera: myths, mechanisms, and management. Blood. 2002;100:4272–90.

Answer to question 27: D

Educational objective

To recognize AML according to the WHO criteria

Critique

In patients with MDS, progression to AML is a risk of the disease and portends a poor prognosis in the majority of patients. The World Health Organization (WHO) classification would classify this patient as having AML. In this situation, consideration should be given to administering AML induction therapy, but this designation of AML is not a mandate for induction chemotherapy. Adult patients with MDS treated with induction chemotherapy typically have lower rates of complete remission, shorter duration of remissions and are more likely to relapse than patients with *de novo* AML. After standard induction chemotherapy, patients are less likely to achieve a complete cytogenetic response, and are more likely to acquire additional cytogenetic abnormalities as the disease progresses.

Decisions regarding the choice of therapy of advanced MDS and MDS progressing to AML are made with several factors in mind. The availability of a suitable donor for a full or mini-transplant, as well as performance status, comorbid medical conditions and an understanding of the expected outcomes with standard induction chemotherapy all need to be considered prior to the initiation of high-intensity therapy.

References

Harris NL, Jaffe ES, Diebold J, Flandrin G, Muller-Hermelink HK, Vardiman J et al. World Health Organization classification of neoplastic diseases of the hematopoietic and lymphoid tissues: report of the clinical advisory committee meeting. Airlie House, Virginia. J Clin Oncol. 1999;17:3835–49.

National Comprehensive Cancer Network. Clinical Practice Guidelines in Oncology, Vol. 1, 2004.

Answer to question 28: E

Educational objective

To recognize the optimal induction regimen for patients with acute promyelocytic leukemia

Critique

Acute promyelocytic leukemia (APL) has emerged as the most curable of all subtypes of AML. The major advance in this regard has been the introduction of all-*trans* retinoic acid (ATRA), a derivative of vitamin A, which induces leukemic promyelocytes to differentiate into mature granulocytes. Leukemic promyelocytes appear particularly sensitive to the effects of anthracyclines. It has become routine to combine ATRA plus an anthracycline, with or without cytarabine. The usual dosage of daunorubicin ranges between 50 and 60 mg/m^2/day for 3 days. While idarubicin may be equally as effective as daunorubicin when combined with ATRA, there is no established role for arsenic trioxide in induction therapy. Similarly, the role of cytarabine has been called into question. However, there is no role for high-dose cytarabine in induction, either alone or combined with ATRA.

References

Fenaux P, Chastagne C, Chevret S, et al. A randomized comparison of all-*trans* retinoic acid (ATRA) followed by chemotherapy and ATRA plus chemotherapy and the role of maintenance therapy in newly diagnosed acute promyelocytic leukemia. Blood. 1999;94:1192–200.

Fenaux P, Le Delay MC, Castaigne S, et al. Effect of all-*trans* retinoic acid in newly diagnosed acute promyelocytic leukemia: results of a multicenter randomized trial. Blood. 1993;82:3241–9.

Sanz MA, Martin G, Rayon C, et al. A modified AIDA protocol with anthracycline-based consolidation results in high antileukemic efficacy and reduced toxicity in newly diagnosed PML-RARα-positive acute promyelocytic leukemia. Blood. 1999;94:3015–21.

Tallman MS, Andersen JW, Schiffer CA, et al. All-*trans* retinoic acid in acute promyelocytic leukemia. N Engl J Med. 1997;337:1021–8.

Answer to question 29: E

Educational objective

To recognize favorable chromosomal findings in childhood ALL

Critique

Hyperdiploidy is a favorable prognostic factor in childhood ALL. Prognosis is especially good in those children whose blasts have 'high' hyperdiploidy (more than 52 chromosomes). Recent data suggest that triploidy of specific chromosomes is more important than hyperdiploidy *per se*. Despite different treatment strategies, the Children's Oncology Group (COG) and Pediatric Oncology Group (POG) have demonstrated that patients whose blasts are triploid for chromosomes 4, 10 and 17 have an event-free survival of >90%. Hypodiploidy, t(4;11) and t(9;22) are poor prognostic factors.

References

Carroll WL, Bhojwani D, Min D-J, et al. Pediatric acute lymphoblastic leukemia. Hematology. 2003;104–7.

Answer to question 30: B

Educational objective

Treatment options for alkylator-resistant CLL

Critique

Fludarabine provides responses in 46% of CLL patients who fail to respond to chlorambucil. Cyclophosphamide, also an alkylating agent, may provide response in a small proportion of chlorambucil-resistant patients. The anti-CD52 monoclonal antibody alemtuzumab is approved for treatment of fludarabine-refractory CLL, and is typically more effective for treatment of CLL involving blood and marrow than for nodal and splenic disease. Single-agent rituximab provides responses in approximately 25% of relapsed CLL patients, but is more effective when used in combination with fludarabine and fludarabine-based chemotherapy combinations.

References

Keating MJ, Flinn I, Jain V, Binet J-L, Hillmen P, Byrd J, et al. Therapeutic role of alemtuzumab (Campath-1H) in patients who have failed fludarabine: results of a large international study. Blood. 2002;99:3554–61.

Rai KR, Peterson BL, Appelbaum FR, Kolitz J, Elias L, Shepherd L, et al. Fludarabine compared with chlorambucil as primary therapy for chronic lymphocytic leukemia. N Engl J Med. 2000;343:1750–7.

Answer to question 31: C

Educational objective

To recognize the differences in risk for graft-versus-host disease among stem cell sources

Critique

For this patient, the stem cell source with the lowest risk of graft-versus-host disease (GVHD) and sufficient hematopoietic progenitors is to elutriate harvested marrow. While the risks of GVHD may be lower with cord blood as the stem cell source, this is usually not practical for an adult because of the limitations in stem cell numbers and the risk of insufficient hematopoietic progenitors. Elutriation partially depletes T cells from the stem cell product. As T cells are mediators of GVHD, this process reduces the risk of developing GVHD. However, with the reduction in immunologic graft-versus-host activity, there is an increased risk of relapse that must be balanced. Rates of acute and chronic GVHD are higher with mobilized peripheral blood stem cells. This is thought to be caused in part by the higher number of T cells in peripheral blood collections than in marrow harvests. Rates of GVHD are highest in unrelated donor transplants because of minor antigen mismatches.

References

Flowers ME, Parker PM, Johnston LJ, Matos AV, Storer B, Bensinger WI, et al. Comparison of chronic graft-versus-host disease after transplantation of peripheral blood stem cells versus bone marrow in allogeneic recipients: long-term follow-up of a randomized controlled trial. Blood. 2002;100:415–9.

Mohty M, Kuentz M, Michallet M, Bourhis JH, Milpied N, Sutton L, et al. Chronic graft-versus-host disease after allogeneic blood stem cell transplantation: long-term results of a randomized controlled study. Blood. 2002;100:3128–34.

Answer to question 32: A

Educational objective

To manage a patient with a new diagnosis of ITP and moderate thrombocytopenia

Critique

With the advent of routine platelet counts performed with all CBCs (a phenomenon of the last 25 years), the spectrum of idiopathic thrombocytopenic purpura (ITP) has increased remarkably. Asymptomatic patients like this were inapparent when platelet counts were only ordered for suspected thrombocytopenia. This enlarged spectrum of ITP, including many patients with no or minimal symptoms who are incidentally discovered, must be incorporated into the broader concept of this disorder.

In the absence of any gold standard tests to diagnose ITP, the diagnosis can only be based on the observation of thrombocytopenia without other hematologic abnormalities, including no other clinically apparent causes for the thrombocytopenia. The data provided for this patient fulfill these criteria. Also, it is important to recognize that the goal for treatment of ITP is only to prevent bleeding, which is not an issue in this woman with mild thrombocytopenia. Treatment is not indicated in the absence of thrombocytopenia when it poses no hemostatic risk. There should be no risk for spontaneous intracranial hemorrhage with this platelet count. Her platelet count had probably been low for a long time prior to her diagnosis, and her absence of important bleeding is reassuring. Prednisone may be appropriate if the platelet count is <20,000–30,000/μL.

When there are no other hematologic abnormalities apparent on routine blood counts and on examination of the peripheral blood smear, examination of the bone marrow does not provide additional important information. It is unnecessary to routinely carry out a bone marrow examination in the evaluation of a patient with suspected ITP. It is not likely that myelodysplasia will be present in the absence of other peripheral blood abnormalities, especially in a younger patient. If this patient was older (for example, >60 years of age), a bone marrow examination to rule out myelodysplasia might be appropriate.

Other etiologies for thrombocytopenia such as inapparent liver disease with hypersplenism or occult lymphoma may be considered, but in the absence of a suggestive history or physical examination these possibilities warrant no further evaluation. However, an HIV test should be considered in patients with thrombocytopenia who have risk factors for HIV infection.

References

Neylon AJ, Saunders PWG, Howard MR, Proctor SJ, Taylor PRA. Clinically significant newly presenting autoimmune thrombocytopenic purpura in adults: a prospective study of a population-based cohort of 245 patients. Br J Haematol. 2003;122:966–74.

Portielje JEA, Westendorp RGJ, Kluin-Nelemans HC, Brand A. Morbidity and mortality in adults with idiopathic thrombocytopenic purpura. Blood. 2001;97:2549–54.

Answer to question 33: D

Educational objective

To recognize the presentation of an acute hemolytic transfusion reaction

Critique

These dramatic symptoms and signs presenting early in a transfusion represent an acute hemolytic transfusion reaction until proven otherwise. Immediate cessation of the transfusion and prompt evaluation are called for, often while normal saline is being given in an effort to maintain urine flow and prevent severe renal damage. The vast majority of these reactions are caused by incompatibilities involving the ABO system. These are overwhelmingly caused by improper identification of the recipient or through mislabeled samples. Laboratory error in ABO typing has become a rare event through the efforts of laboratory regulatory agencies which require maintenance of staff proficiency and competency as well as quality control systems for sample processing and reporting results. Antibodies with specificity for the A and B antigens occur naturally and are expected to be present in antigen-negative individuals. These antibodies are always of the IgM class and, although reactive at colder temperatures like most IgM antibodies, making their detection at room temperature possible, they bind to antigen-positive red cells at 37°C. This leads to a rapid onset of intravascular hemolysis and activation of complement and other inflammatory cascades, releasing vasoactive peptides. The symptoms experienced by this patient may overlap with other adverse reactions that can present early in transfusion, but the red urine is a clue that intravascular hemolysis is present. Rh antibodies rarely fix complement and cause chiefly extravascular hemolysis, with a paucity of most other symptoms. Besides, Rh-negative blood lacks the RhD antigen, and can safely be given to Rh-positive individuals. Bacterial contamination is commonly associated with platelet products, which must be stored at 22°C rather than in the refrigerator like red cell units. Storage under refrigerated conditions keeps the incidence of reactions to contaminated red cells extremely low. Although cytokine-mediated reactions may present early in transfusion and cause some overlapping symptoms, especially fever and hypotension, they are not associated with hemolysis.

References

Deb B, Wendling WW, Mintz P, Levin R, Manno CS, Herman JH. A non-fatal acute hemolytic transfusion reaction in a young trauma victim. Am J Anesthesiol. 1998;25:31–3.

Sazama K. Transfusion errors: scope of the problem, consequences, and solutions. Curr Hematol Rep. 2003;2:518–21.

Answer to question 34: C

Educational objective

To diagnose von Willebrand disease

Critique

von Willebrand disease is the most common inherited bleeding disorder and usually presents with bleeding from mucosal surfaces; the family history indicates an autosomal dominant inheritance. Factor XI deficiency is an autosomal recessive disease and is much less common statistically. A bleeding time would be nonspecific if it was abnormal, and platelet aggregation studies would test for an intrinsic platelet disorder, a much less common inherited disease. Electron microscopy is usually performed for intrinsic platelet disorders after other testing indicates a likelihood of a platelet disorder, such as in platelet storage pool disease.

References

Bevan JA, Maloney KW, Hillery CA, Gill JC, Montgomery RR, Scott JP. Bleeding disorders: a common cause of menorrhagia in adolescents. J Pediatr. 2001;138:856–61.

Kadir RA, Aledort LM. Obstetrical and gynaecological bleeding: a common presenting symptom. Clin Lab Haematol. 2000;22(Suppl.1):12–6; discussion 30–2.

Answer to question 35: C

Educational objective

To prescribe DVT prophylaxis in a patient undergoing knee replacement therapy

Critique

Without prophylaxis, deep vein thrombosis (DVT) occurs in approximately 50% of healthy patients after hip or knee replacement. Because DVT can lead to fatal pulmonary embolism and chronic postphlebitic syndrome, prophylaxis is strongly advised regardless of a history of thrombophilia. In addition, these tests would not be appropriate for a man who had his first and only DVT at age 71 and whose DVT was related to a surgical procedure. The choice of therapeutic agent is a matter of preference unless the patient has contraindications to one of the agents. Three popular agents are LMWH, warfarin and fondaparinux. LMWH is associated with a lower thrombotic rate but somewhat higher bleeding risk when compared with warfarin; fondaparinux is associated with a lower thrombotic rate (12.5% versus 27%) but greater bleeding risk (2.7% versus 1.5%) when compared with LMWH. Recent studies suggest further benefit if prophylaxis is continued for 10 days or more, even after the patient is ambulatory and discharged. Although any of the three agents would be a correct answer to the question, only LMWH was offered as an option. Currently, the choice is based on practitioner experience and cost considerations. Aspirin and dextran are inferior to LMWH, warfarin or fondaparinux in this setting. Graded compression stockings and early ambulation are of no proven benefit.

References

Bauer KA, Eriksson BI, Lassen MR, Turpie AG, Steering Committee of the Pentasaccharide in Major Knee Surgery Study. Fondaparinux compared with enoxaparin for the prevention of venous thromboembolism after elective major knee surgery. N Engl J Med. 2001;345:1305–10.

Geerts WH, Heit JA, Clagett GP, Pineo GF, Colwell CW, Anderson FA, et al. Prevention of venous thromboembolism. Chest. 2001;119(Suppl):132.

Answer to question 36: A

Educational objective

To evaluate a patient for relapsed CML after stem cell transplantation

Critique

Because RT-PCR studies are so sensitive, the results must be interpreted with caution. Miniscule levels of contamination can yield false-positive results. All PCR assays should have appropriate positive and negative controls. The clinical significance of a single positive RT-PCR result after prior negative results is unclear. Serial quantitative RT-PCR studies that show rising levels of positivity predict relapse and may prompt medical intervention.

References

Eder M, Battmer K, Kafert S, Stucki A, Ganser A, Hertenstein B. Monitoring of BCR-ABL expression using real-time RT-PCR in CML after bone marrow or peripheral blood stem cell transplantation. Leukemia. 1999;13:1383–9.

Miyamura K, Tahara T, Tanimoto M, Morishita Y, Kawashima K, Morishima Y, et al. Long persistent *bcr-abl* positive transcript detected by polymerase chain reaction after marrow transplant from chronic myelogenous leukemia without clinical relapse: a study of 64 patients. Blood. 1993;81:1089–93.

Answer to question 37: D

Educational objective

To treat Fanconi anemia and bone marrow failure

Critique

This patient has Fanconi anemia with severe bone marrow failure. Stem cell transplantation is the best treatment. However, the cellular hypersensitivity of these patients to alkylating agents such as cyclophosphamide and irradiation has led to attenuated dose regimens with a demonstrated reduction in acute toxicity. Although these attenuated dose conditioning regimens are preferred, the numbers of patients available for study are small and the ideal conditioning regimen for aplastic anemia in these patients has not been definitively identified. This is even more true for the Fanconi anemia patient with myelodysplastic syndrome. In addition to increased conditioning-related toxicity, patients with Fanconi anemia are at increased risk for graft-versus-host disease and its complications. However, stem cell transplant is the only treatment option that corrects the hematological manifestations of this disease.

Immunosuppression is usually not effective in relieving the cytopenias associated with Fanconi anemia.

Induction chemotherapy is not indicated for this patient who does not have acute myeloid leukemia.

References

Deeg HJ, Socie G, Schoch G, Henry-Amar M, Witherspoon RP, Devergie A, et al. Malignancies after marrow transplantation for aplastic anemia: a joint Seattle and Paris analysis of results of 700 patients. Blood. 1996;87:386–92.

Dufour C, Rondelli D, Locatelli F, et al. Stem cell transplantation from HLA-matched related donor for Fanconi anemia: a retrospective review of the multicentric Italian experience on behalf of AIEOP-GITMO. Br J Haematol. 2001;112:796–805.

Answer to question 38: D

Educational objective

To treat chemotherapy-associated anemia

Critique

This patient has fatigue and hemoglobin of approximately 9 g/dL. The ASH/ASCO guidelines suggest treatment of chemotherapy-induced anemia if the hemoglobin is ≤10 g/dL to improve symptoms and quality of life. It is not necessary to transfuse PRBC, as there is no urgent need to increase his HCT. Darbepoetin alfa, which has a much longer half-life *in vivo* than epoetin alfa, effectively increases the HCT when given once per chemotherapy cycle. Epoetin alfa is also effective for chemotherapy-induced anemia, but is usually administered once weekly or more frequently.

Reference

Rizzo JD, et al. Use of epoetin in patients with cancer: evidence-based clinical practice guidelines of the American Society of Clinical Oncology and the American Society of Hematology. Blood. 2002;100:2303–20.

Answer to question 39: A

Educational objective

To recognize the protein that is a mediator of the anemia of chronic inflammation

Critique

Iron absorption is a complicated process that is not completely understood. Recently, hepcidin, a naturally occurring antimicrobial peptide, has been shown to be a major regulator of iron hemostasis and to likely be the key mediator of the anemia of inflammation. Hepcidin is made in the liver and its transcription is strongly induced by interleukin-6 (IL-6). Hepcidin synthesis is down-regulated in iron-deficient states. Hepcidin has been shown to impair macrophage iron recycling and intestinal iron absorption, producing a picture consistent with the anemia of inflammation. Recently, patients with hepatic adenomas have been shown to have high tissue expression of hepcidin and to have resolution of anemia following resection of the adenomas. HFE and DMT1 are both membrane-associated proteins in the intestinal crypt cell that facilitate iron absorption. Hephestin and ceruloplasmin arc ferroxidases that are also membrane bound and act to convert Fe^{2+} to Fe^{3+} such that transferrin binding can occur.

References

Ganz T. Hepcidin, a key regulator of iron metabolism and mediator of anemia of inflammation. Blood. 2003;102:783–8.

Weinstein DA, Roy CN, Fleming MD, Loda MF, Wolfsdorf JI, Andrews NC. Inappropriate expression of hepcidin is associated with iron refractory anemia: implications for the anemia of chronic disease. Blood. 2002;100:3776–81.

Answer to question 40: E

Educational objective

To recognize alternative intravenous iron preparations for patients with allergy to iron dextran

Critique

Iron sucrose is the most widely used hematinic worldwide. It can be safely given in doses of 100 mg over several minutes. It has a markedly low incidence of anaphylactic reactions and can be used safely in patients who are intolerant to iron dextran. Nonlife-threatening reactions including hypotension, rash and nausea are extremely uncommon. Dialysis patients have extremely high iron requirements and the patient in question has intermittent gastrointestinal blood loss. Oral iron replacement would not be effective in promoting erythropoietin-dependent erythropoiesis in this patient. Neither histamine receptor antagonists nor glucocorticoids can be expected to reliably prevent anaphylaxis in patients allergic to iron dextran.

Reference

Yed J, Besarab A. Iron sucrose: the oldest iron therapy becomes new. Am J Kidney Dis. 2002;40:1111–21.

Answer to question 41: A

Educational objective

To recognize the clinical presentation and laboratory evaluation of paroxysmal nocturnal hemoglobinuria

Critique

This patient has a prior history of aplastic anemia and is now found to have pancytopenia and newly diagnosed Budd–Chiari syndrome. Paroxysmal nocturnal hemoglobinuria (PNH) should be suspected based both on its known association with aplastic anemia and other primary bone marrow disorders, as well as with hepatic vein occlusion. Previously, the diagnosis of PNH was made by the Ham test or sucrose hemolysis test, but currently is typically diagnosed by the absence of the glycosyl phosphatidylinositol (GPI)-anchored proteins, CD59 or CD55, expressed on the surface of red blood cells or leukocytes. The occurrence of factor V Leiden would not explain the cytopenias and is rarely associated with hepatic vein occlusion in the heterozygous and even homozygous state. Analysis of BFU-E should be considered if polycythemia vera was the likely diagnosis and the test could be arranged at a referral center. Deficiency of vitamin B_{12} may cause pancytopenia, but would not explain hepatic vein occlusion.

References

Dunn DE, Tanawattanacharoen P, Boccuni P, Nagakura S, Green SW, Kirby MR, et al. Paroxysmal nocturnal hemoglobinuria cells in patients with bone marrow failure syndromes. Ann Intern Med. 1999;131:401–8.

Rosse WF. Paroxysmal nocturnal hemoglobinuria as a molecular disease. Medicine (Baltimore). 1997;76:63–93.

Answer to question 42: B

Educational objective

To recognize the clinicopathologic features of familial Mediterranean fever

Critique

Collectively, this patient's ethnic background and long-standing history of unexplained fever and inflammatory episodes with neutrophilia, synovitis, lymphadenopathy and mild splenomegaly are highly suggestive of familial Mediterranean fever (FMF). Proteinuria and elevated creatinine are consistent with renal AA amyloidosis, a major long-term complication in adults with poorly controlled FMF. Further investigation of family history will likely identify similarly affected siblings or other relatives. FMF is an autosomal recessive disorder caused by mutations in the *MEFV* gene. *MEFV* encodes the myeloid-specific protein pyrin, which is believed to function by down-modulating neutrophil inflammatory responses. Symptoms of FMF usually begin in childhood but may go unrecognized or undiagnosed for many years. Clinical manifestations and end-organ complications of AA amyloidosis are usually controlled or prevented by colchicine. Although some of the clinical and/or laboratory features of this case may suggest gout due to chronic myeloid leukemia (CML; associated with the *BCR-ABL* gene rearrangement), systemic mastocytosis (which is often associated with an Asp-816-Val c-*kit* point mutation) or low-grade non-Hodgkin lymphoma (associated with the *IgH-BCL2* gene rearrangement), those acquired disorders would not have the lifelong history and are not associated with inflammatory episodes and nephrotic syndrome. The familial variant of hemophagocytic lymphohistiocytosis (FHLH; associated with mutations involving the perforin gene, *PRF1*) commonly presents as a severe aggressive multisystem disorder in early childhood. Therefore, it would not be a consideration in this adult patient.

References

Samuels J, Aksentijevich I, Torosyan Y, Centola M, Deng Z, Sood R, et al. Familial Mediterranean fever at the millennium: clinical spectrum, ancient mutations, and a survey of 100 American referrals to the National Institutes of Health. Medicine (Baltimore). 1998;77:268–97.

Tidow N, Chen X, Muller C, Kawano S, Gombart AF, Fischel-Ghodsian N, et al. Hematopoietic-specific expression of *MEFV*, the gene mutated in familial Mediterranean fever, and subcellular localization of its corresponding protein, pyrin. Blood. 2000;95:1451–5.

Tuglular S, Yalcinkaya F, Paydas S, Oner A, Utas C, Bozfakioglu S, et al. A retrospective analysis for aetiology and clinical findings of 287 secondary amyloidosis cases in Turkey. Nephrol Dial Transplant. 2002;17:2003–5.

Answer to question 43: B

Educational objective

To recognize the prognosis of MDS with 5q- as the sole cytogenetic abnormality

Critique

Patients with MDS and cytogenetic studies showing 5q- as the only abnormality have a unique clinical picture and prognosis. They are less likely to progress to overt AML, and typically present with only anemia. The platelet count is usually normal or sometimes increased. Given their relatively good prognosis compared with other forms of MDS, careful consideration should be given prior to proceeding with higher intensity therapies. The majority of these patients are managed with close monitoring and supportive care. Intensive chemotherapeutic approaches should only be considered after patients have failed less intense treatment approaches including growth factor support, and have demonstrated progression of their disease in terms of transfusion requirements and increases in bone marrow blast percentages. Thrombocytosis is one of the clinical features seen in the 5q-syndrome.

Therapy of the thrombocytosis is not indicated and could expose the patient to side-effects without any clear clinical benefit.

References

Giagounidis AAN, Germing U, Haase S, Hildebrandt B, Schlegelberger B, Schoch C et al. Clinical, morphological, cytogenetic, and prognostic features of patients with myelodysplastic syndromes and del (5q) including band q31. Leukemia. 2004;18:113–9.

Mathew P, Tefferi A, Dewald GW, Goldberg SL, Su J, Hoagland HC, et al. The 5q- syndrome: a single-institution study of 43 consecutive patients. Blood. 1993;81:1040–5.

Answer to question 44: B

Educational objective

To understand the beneficial effect of hematopoietic growth factors during induction therapy in patients with AML

Critique

The hematopoietic growth factors are glycoproteins that stimulate the proliferation, differentiation and maturation of hematopoietic cells. It had initially been hoped that they would improve outcome in patients with AML when given during induction. However, multiple studies have now shown that the complete remission rate is not improved. Similarly, overall survival is not improved. However, the duration of neutropenia is reduced and there appears to be little risk of stimulation of leukemic cells. Although some studies have shown a reduction in induction mortality and less fungal infection, they have not eliminated the risk of gram-negative bacteremia.

References

Dombret H, Chastagne C, Fenaux P, et al. A controlled study of recombinant human granulocyte colony-stimulating factor in elderly patients after treatment for acute myelogenous leukemia.

AML Cooperative Study Group. N Engl J Med. 1995;332:1678–83.

Godwin JE, Kopecky KJ, Head DR, et al. A double-blind placebo-controlled trial of granulocyte colony-stimulating factor in elderly patients with previously untreated acute myeloid leukemia: a Southwest Oncology Group Study (9031). Blood. 1998;91:3607–15.

Lowenberg B, Suciu S, Archimbaud E, et al. Use of recombinant GM-CSF during and after remission induction chemotherapy in patients aged 61 years and older with acute myeloid leukemia: final report of AML-11, a phase III randomized study of the Leukemia Cooperative Group of the European Organization for Research and Treatment of Cancer and the Dutch–Belgium Hemato-Oncology Cooperative Group. Blood. 1997;90:2952–61.

Answer to question 45: C

Educational objective

To recognize prognostic factors and IPI score in aggressive B-cell lymphoma

Critique

The International Prognostic Index (IPI) score utilizes five clinical parameters—age >60 years, stage III or IV, performance status of 2–4, elevated LDH and two or more sites of extranodal disease—to assign a prognostic score in large cell and other lymphomas. This patient's score of two (stage, PS) places her in a low–intermediate risk group with a predicted 5-year survival of 51% with anthracycline-based chemotherapy. The addition of rituximab to CHOP increased the 3-year overall survival versus CHOP alone in the French GELA study in patients above the age of 60 years, but the impact on 5-year survival is as yet uncertain.

References

Coiffier B, Lepage E, Briere J, Herbrecht R, Tilly H, Bouabdallah R, et al. CHOP chemotherapy plus rituximab compared with CHOP alone in elderly patients with diffuse large B-cell lymphoma. N Engl J Med. 2002;346:235–42.

Shipp MA. Prognostic factors in aggressive non-Hodgkin lymphoma: who has 'high-risk' disease? Blood. 1994;83:1165–73.

Answer to question 46: D

Educational objective

To recognize the indications for nonmyeloablative allogeneic stem cell transplant

Critique

The optimal transplantation for this patient, if he is going to receive one, is a nonmyeloablative allogeneic transplant. The reasons for this are several-fold. First, this patient has received a total of 20 cycles of chemotherapy prior to being evaluated and is considered to be heavily pretreated. When the number of cycles of therapy exceeds 12, the risks of morbidity and mortality rise with myeloablative preparative regimens. Further, it is more difficult to mobilize stem cells in this population because of prior chemotherapy, making autologous transplant difficult. At age 63 years, he is considered too old by most centers for a myeloablative allogeneic transplant because of the risks of morbidity and mortality following the procedure. His disease, while incurable with standard chemotherapy, may be eradicated through immunologic means of graft-versus-host responses. Thus, a non-myeloablative allogeneic transplant that employs reduced intensity conditioning regimens followed by allogeneic stem cells has the potential to induce an immunologic antitumor effect in this patient. Although he is in complete remission now, his disease will recur and so the first option is incorrect.

References

Baron F, Beguin Y. Nonmyeloablative allogeneic hematopoietic stem cell transplantation. J Hematother Stem Cell Res. 2002;11:243–63.

Shimoni A, Nagler A. Non-myeloablative hematopoietic stem cell transplantation (NST) in the treatment of human malignancies: from animal models to clinical practice. Cancer Treat Res. 2002;110:113–36.

Answer to question 47: A

Educational objective

To recognize favorable prognostic factors in childhood ALL

Critique

Complete remission is achieved by 98–99% of children with ALL using three- or four-drug treatment. Remission rates are highest (99%) in patients with standard risk ALL (age 1–9 years) and WBC ≤50,000/μL. Patients with higher risk ALL (age >9 years or WBC >50,000/μL) have a lower remission rate (98%) as do infants (90–95%), patients with T-cell ALL (90–95%) and patients with a t(9;22) (85–90%). Pretreatment with corticosteroids prior to the diagnosis of ALL also decreases the rate of achieving complete remission, although a rapid response to 1 week of prednisone given after the ALL diagnosis is a favorable prognostic finding.

References

Arico M, Valsecchi MG, Camitta B, et al. Outcome of treatment in children with Philadelphia chromosome-positive acute lymphoblastic leukemia. N Engl J Med. 2000;342:998–1006.

Silverman LB, Gelber RD, Young ML, et al. Induction failure in acute lymphoblastic leukemia of childhood. Cancer. 1999;85:1395–404.

Answer to question 48: D

Educational objective

To recognize transfusion-acquired graft-versus-host disease

Critique

Transfusion-induced graft-versus-host disease (GVHD) is caused by immunocompetent donor lymphocytes that mount an antihost response, often within 1–3 weeks after transfusion, and shares many features with GVHD after allogeneic stem cell transplantation. The chief difference is that the hematopoietic cells in post-transplant GVHD are of donor origin, and so marrow function is often preserved, while transfusion-induced GVHD causes profound pancytopenia as hematopoiesis fails. This accounts for the high fatality rate of transfusion-induced GVHD. Although there is a theoretical threshold of lymphocyte exposure below which there is minimal risk, currently available leukoreduction and pathogen inactivation technologies have not been validated to prevent transfusion-induced GVHD. Prevention depends on gamma irradiation of all cellular components to render donor lymphocytes incapable of mounting an antihost response. There is no consensus regarding all the patient groups at risk for transfusion-induced GVHD, but most centers agree that fetuses and premature infants, and patients with congenital combined or T-cell immune deficiencies, aplastic anemia and Hodgkin lymphoma require GVHD prophylaxis, and many include all patients with acute leukemia. Directed donation from close blood relatives, or from donors in ethnic populations with a limited repertoire of HLA types, can lead to haplo-identical donor lymphocytes being transfused and causing GVHD. It has recently been shown that fludarabine itself, even when given outside the setting of CLL or lymphoid malignancy, can lead to transfusion-induced GVHD. While CLL is also associated with a number of immune cytopenias, the other symptoms are the classic triad of GVHD. Systemic CMV infection can cause gastrointestinal disease, a rash and lower blood counts, but the majority of CMV reactivations in CLL patients cause organ-specific problems or herpes zoster. Fludarabine toxicity may cause some of these findings, but is not this severe and resolves after a week or two. CLL is certainly at risk for transformation to high-grade lymphoma, but again the combination of the presenting symptoms is not characteristic of this.

References

Leitman SF, Tisdale JF, Bolan CD, Popovsky MA, Klippel JH, Balow JE, et al. Transfusion-associated GVHD after fludarabine therapy in a patient with systemic lupus erythematosus. Transfusion. 2003;43:1667–71.

Maung ZT, Wood AC, Jackson GH, Turner GE, Appleton AL, Hamilton PJ. Transfusion-associated graft-versus-host disease in fludarabine-treated B-chronic lymphocytic leukaemia. Br J Haematol. 1995;88:649–52.

Przepiorka D, LeParc GF, Stovall MA, Werch J, Lichtiger B. Use of irradiated blood components: practice parameter. Am J Clin Pathol. 1996;106:6–11.

Answer to question 49: C

Educational objective

To evaluate a patient for a congenital bleeding disorder who presents with normal coagulation screening studies

Critique

The normal screening studies for the coagulation cascade, for von Willebrand disease and for platelet function suggest that this patient has another deficiency that does not affect these assays. α_2-Antiplasmin deficiency, factor XIII deficiency and plasminogen activator inhibitor-1 (PAI-1) deficiency are possible causes for bleeding that do not give abnormal screening assays. Platelet aggregation studies are less likely to be helpful in the face of normal platelet function analyzer studies, immunologic fibrinogen is not indicated because the thrombin time is normal, and a decreased factor XII would give a prolonged APTT. Examining the peripheral smear, while important, would not be most helpful in determining the reason for bleeding in this patient.

References

Miles LA, Plow EF, Donnelly KJ, Hougie C, Griffin JH. A bleeding disorder due to deficiency of α_2-antiplasmin. Blood. 1982;59:1246–51.

Saito H. α_2-Plasmin inhibitor and its deficiency states. J Lab Clin Med. 1988;112:671–8.

Answer to question 50: B

Educational objective

To evaluate a patient with a bleeding disorder

Critique

The donor's history suggests a hereditary bleeding disorder but is inconclusive. A history of menorrhagia is subjective and difficult to quantify. The postoperative bleeding could have related to a surgical error rather than a systemic disorder, but the history of major blood loss combined with a maternal history of bleeding increase the likelihood that the patient has a hereditary bleeding diathesis. In addition, she is about to undergo an elective procedure for which the risk of severe bleeding justifies a thorough evaluation. A bleeding time is not useful in predicting perioperative bleeding and is a poor screening test. von Willebrand disease is a common hereditary bleeding diathesis in people of European descent (1 in 1000), is often manifested by menorrhagia and severe bleeding following surgery without other evidence of a hemorrhagic diathesis, and may be associated with a normal APTT even if factor VIII is deficient. It is inherited as an autosomal dominant trait. Factor XI deficiency, relatively rare in all but Ashkenazi Jews, is usually associated with an elevated APTT and with slow oozing following minor surgery on mucous membranes (ENT, GU) rather than brisk bleeding after organ removal. Factor XI deficiency is inherited as an autosomal recessive disorder although heterozygotes may be symptomatic. Similarly, dysfibrino-genemia is a relatively rare cause of bleeding. Of note, if the patient is found to have a hereditary bleeding diathesis, her daughter should also be evaluated for the disorder prior to transplant surgery.

Reference

Sadler JE. Von Willebrand disease type 1: a diagnosis in search of a disease. Blood. 2003;101:2089–93.

Answer to question 51: C

Educational objective

To detect the factor V Leiden point mutation in a young patient with deep venous thrombosis

Critique

Most patients with APC resistance carry the factor V Leiden mutation, in which a mutation in factor V destroys the major site at which protein C cleaves and inactivates factor Va. This mutation destroys a recognition site for the enzyme MnlI, allowing for rapid diagnosis of the factor V Leiden mutation. Oligonucleotides flanking the factor V cleavage site are used to amplify the target region by PCR, and the resultant PCR products are digested with MnlI. DNA amplified from patients with the mutation will not digest with MnlI, yielding a larger (undigested) fragment after restriction enzyme digestion. Diagnosis of heterozygous or homozygous factor V Leiden mutation is then made by detection of this larger fragment by agarose gel electrophoresis. In this clinical entity, there is not an abnormality in the protein C gene. Therefore, Southern blot analysis of the protein C gene is not diagnostically useful. Because factor V is not a protein that is expressed by blood cells, RT-PCR of peripheral blood would not be the method of choice for demonstrating the mutation. The factor V Leiden mutation accounts for the vast majority of cases of APC resistance. If the factor V Leiden mutation were not detected in a patient with APC resistance, family linkage analysis may help elucidate the molecular basis.

References

Bertina RM, Koeleman BP, Koster T, Rosendaal FR, Dirven RJ, de Ronde H, et al. Mutation in blood coagulation factor V associated with resistance to activated protein C. Nature. 1994;369:64–7.

Juul K, Tybjaerg-Hansen A, Schnohr P, Nordestgaard BG. Factor V Leiden and the risk for venous thromboembolism in the adult Danish population. Ann Intern Med. 2004;140:330–7.

Answer to question 52: D

Educational objective

To identify Fanconi anemia as a cause of myelodysplastic syndrome in a pediatric patient

Critique

The question pertains to a Fanconi anemia patient with myelodysplastic syndrome.

The prevalence of acute myeloid leukemia (AML) and myelodysplastic syndrome in Fanconi anemia is substantially increased and has been estimated to be 15,000 times higher than that in the general population. The incidence of myelodysplasia and AML in these patients increases with age, occurring on average 10 years from the initial diagnosis of hematologic abnormalities. Some patients may present with AML as the initial diagnosis without a known preceding myelodysplastic phase. Although AML has been reported with the other causes of inherited bone marrow failure (dyskeratosis congenita, Shcwachman–Diamond syndrome, amegakaryocytic thrombocytopenia), the increased risk is not as great as it is with Fanconi anemia. Also, these other disorders do not demonstrate the chromosomal fragility and sensitivity to clastogenic agents seen in Fanconi anemia.

Reference

Sieff CA, Nisbet-Brown E, Nathan D. Congenital bone marrow failure syndromes. Br J Haematol. 2000;111:30–42.

Answer to question 53: D

Educational objective

To recognize the clinical effects of filgrastim therapy in peripheral blood stem cell transplantation

Critique

Following chemotherapy, filgrastim effectively mobilizes increased numbers of $CD34^+$ peripheral blood progenitor cells and/or stem cells, which lead to more rapid engraftment in both autologous and allogeneic transplantation. Filgrastim administered post-transplant is not necessary when peripheral blood stem cells are used in the transplant procedure. Side-effects attributable to filgrastim are usually mild and manageable with conventional analgesics. No increased incidence of acute graft-versus-host disease has been seen with filgrastim-mobilized allografts. Although granulocyte recovery is more rapid with mobilized peripheral blood stem cells, overall mortality is not improved.

References

Bensinger WI, Martin PJ, Storer B, Clift R, Forman SJ, Negrin R, et al. Transplantation of bone marrow as compared with peripheral-blood cells from HLA-identical relatives in patients with hematologic cancers. N Engl J Med. 2001;344:175–81.

Ho VT, Mirza NQ, Junco Dd D, Okamura T, Przepiorka D. The effect of hematopoietic growth factors on the risk of graft-versus-host disease after allogeneic hematopoietic stem cell transplantation: a meta-analysis. Bone Marrow Transplant. 2003;32:771–5.

Maloney DG, Molina AJ, Sahebi F, Stockerl-Goldstein KE, Sandmaier BM, Bensinger W, et al. Allografting with nonmyeloablative conditioning following cytoreductive autografts for the treatment of patients with multiple myeloma. Blood. 2003;102:3447–54.

Answer to question 54: E

Educational objective

To recognize the prognosis in an asymptomatic patient with hereditary hemochromatosis

Critique

This patient was diagnosed with homozygous hemochromatosis based on genetic screening. She is currently asymptomatic, not iron overloaded and does not consume alcohol. Serial ferritin values should be followed throughout life to monitor for early laboratory evidence of iron overload as the clinical penetrance of homozygous hereditary hemochromatosis is uncertain, but likely lower than previously thought. It is therefore incorrect to state that she will definitively develop iron overload later in life. All offspring will inherit one *C282Y* gene from the mother. However, as this mutation is common in the Caucasian population, offspring may also inherit a C282Y mutation from the father, if he is a carrier. It is therefore premature to state that all children will be heterozygous for the C282Y mutation. If ferritin levels do not become elevated, phlebotomy will not be necessary. Screening for hepatoma should be considered only if there is evidence of cirrhosis.

References

Ajioka RS, Kushner JP. Clinical consequences of iron overload in hemochromatosis homozygotes. Blood. 2003;101:3351–3.

Beutler E. The HFE Cys282Tyr mutation as a necessary but not sufficient cause of clinical hereditary hemochromatosis. Blood. 2003;101:3347–50.

Harrison SA, Bacon BR. Hereditary hemochromatosis: update for 2003. J Hepatol. 2003;38(Suppl.1):S14–23.

Answer to question 55: C

Educational objective

To treat erythropoietin hyporesponsive anemia in an iron-overloaded patient

Critique

Adequate utilizable iron is essential for normal response to supplemental erythropoietin in dialysis patients. The most common cause of hyporesponsiveness to erythropoietin is lack of available iron, even in patients with apparent iron overload. Iron supplementation is not indicated for patients with biochemical evidence of iron overload. Ascorbic acid can potentiate the mobilization of iron from inert tissue stores and facilitates the incorporation of iron into protoporphyrin in iron-overloaded dialysis patients being treated with erythropoietin. Darbepoetin is an analog of erythropoietin that has increased receptor affinity and can therefore be given on a less frequent dosing regimen. As with erythropoietin, utilizable iron is needed for erythropoiesis in patients receiving darbepoetin. Iron chelation will not improve anemia in this patient as iron is necessary for erythropoiesis.

References

Lin CL, Hsu PY, Yang HY, Huang CC. Low dose intravenous ascorbic acid for erythropoietin-hyporesponsive anemia in diabetic hemodialysis patients with iron overload. Ren Fail. 2003;25:445–53.

Tarng DC, Huang TP, Wei YH. Erythropoietin and iron: the role of ascorbic acid. Nephrol Dial Transplant. 2001;16(Suppl.5):35–9.

Answer to question 56: B

Educational objective

To diagnose hemoglobin S-β^+ thalassemia

Critique

This patient has a mild microcytic anemia, hemoglobin S and an elevated hemoglobin A_2 documented on hemoglobin electrophoresis. His mother with microcytic anemia likely has β^+ thalassemia and his father, who has a normal hemoglobin level, most likely has sickle cell trait. The patient, based on his blood counts and hemoglobin electrophoretic pattern, has S-β^+ thalassemia. Sickle cell trait can be ruled out by the presence of anemia and the greater percentage of Hb S than Hb A on electrophoresis. S-β° thalassemia can be ruled out given the mild symptoms and the presence of Hb A. Hb SS-hereditary persistence of fetal hemoglobin is ruled out both by the presence of Hb A and because the Hb F level is below 20%. Sickled erythrocytes may be few in number or absent on the peripheral blood smear in S-β^+ thalassemia.

References

NIH Publication no. 02–2117. The Management of Sickle Cell Disease, 4th edn. June 2002:9.

Weatherall DJ. The thalassemias. In: Beutler E, Lichtman MA, Coller BS, Kipps TJ, Seligsohn U, eds. Williams Hematology, 6th edn. New York: McGraw-Hill, 2001:547–80.

Answer to question 57: B

Educational objective

To recognize the clinicopathologic features, diagnostic considerations and management approaches in patients with secondary hemophagocytic lymphohistiocytosis

Critique

Secondary hemophagocytic lymphohistiocytosis (SHLH) should be suspected in patients with unexplained multiorgan dysfunction syndrome, rapidly progressive cytopenias, liver abnormalities and hypofibrinogenemia in the setting of underlying immune dysregulation (e.g. systemic lupus erythematosus), acquired immunouppression, infections or malignancy. SHLH is characterized by activation of histiocytes, cytotoxic T lymphocytes and, in some cases, natural killer cells leading to tissue infiltration and injury. Cytophagic histiocytes, which are primarily responsible for the pancytopenia, may be found in the marrow, lymph nodes, spleen and other tissues. In this case, the marrow hemophagocytic histiocytes point to SHLH as a major pathogenic process; however, the underlying primary cause, which might be an opportunistic infection or occult malignancy (e.g. non-Hodgkin lymphoma), still needs to be determined. The triggering disorder must be appropriately diagnosed and effectively treated to avoid the 40–60% mortality associated with SHLH. A lymph node biopsy, with studies to identify reactive versus malignant B, T or NK cells, and special assays for bacteria, fungi, viruses or atypical organisms, would be the most informative and important next step in the management of this patient. In the absence of lymphadenopathy, further special studies on the marrow, blood, lung tissue or bronchoalveolar lavage fluid may be required to assess for infection or malignancy. Cyclophosphamide would be an appropriate treatment in the setting of an acute severe flare of systemic lupus, catastrophic antiphospholipid syndrome or proven lymphoma; however, this agent would be detrimental if the patient had an underlying opportunistic infection. Similarly, plasma exchange would be helpful for thrombotic thrombocytopenic purpura (TTP) or possibly for severe lupus-related syndromes but would not be indicated otherwise. Ganciclovir might benefit a patient with systemic Epstein–Barr virus or cytomegalovirus infection; however, the myelosuppressive side-effect of this drug makes it a risky choice for empirical therapy. Etoposide, cyclophosphamide, plasma exchange, cyclosporine A and intravenous immunoglobulin have been used adjunctively in patients with unresponsive or progressive SHLH in the setting of infections, malignancies or autoimmune diseases. Those modalities are also used for 'idiopathic' SHLH when an underlying precipitating cause cannot be found.

References

Dhote R, Simon J, Papo T, Detournay B, Sailler L, Andre MH, et al. Reactive hemophagocytic syndrome in adult systemic disease: report of twenty-six cases and literature review. Arthritis Rheum. 2003;49:633–9.

Gauvin F, Toledano B, Champagne J, Lacroix J. Reactive hemophagocytic syndrome presenting as a component of multiple organ dysfunction syndrome. Crit Care Med. 2000;28:3341–5.

Imashuku S, Kuriyama K, Sakai R, Nakao Y, Masuda S, Yasuda N, et al. Treatment of Epstein–Barr virus-associated hemophagocytic lymphohistiocytosis (EBV-HLH) in young adults: a report from the HLH study center. Med Pediatr Oncol. 2003;41:103–9.

Answer to question 58: E

Educational objective

To differentiate essential thrombocythemia and chronic idiopathic myelofibrosis

Critique

The differential diagnosis in this case includes reactive or secondary causes of thrombocytosis, due to iron deficiency, bleeding, infection and inflammation, and myeloproliferative disorder (MPD). The increased platelet count in MPDs is caused by inappropriate autonomous overproduction. Among the MPDs, essential thrombocythemia (ET) is characterized by thrombocytosis in the absence of a secondary cause and without clinicopathologic features of polycythemia vera, idiopathic myelofibrosis (IMF) or chronic myeloid leukemia. Thrombocytosis along with platelet function defects (as revealed by platelet aggregation studies), splenomegaly and marrow hypercellularity with megakaryocyte clustering may be seen with any of the MPDs. Therefore, additional peripheral blood, marrow or cytogenetic abnormalities must be sought to discriminate ET from the other MPDs. The finding of significant marrow reticulin fibrosis and prominent blood leukoerythroblastic features in this patient is more indicative of early fibrotic IMF, and not typical of ET. These features are important because the median survival with early-stage IMF is 10.5 years (with inevitable disease progression and complications over time), whereas the life expectancy with ET can be normal if thrombotic and bleeding complications are avoided.

References

Harrison CN, Green AR. Essential thrombocythemia. Hematol Oncol Clin North Am. 2003;17:1175–90.

Thiele J, Kvasnicka HM. Chronic myeloproliferative disorders with thrombocythemia: a comparative study of two classification systems (PVSG, WHO) on 839 patients. Ann Hematol. 2003;82:148–52.

Answer to question 59: C

Educational objective

To differentiate aplastic anemia from the hypocellular form of MDS

Critique

Up to 20% of patients with MDS may present with a hypocellular bone marrow. In practice, it may be quite difficult to differentiate aplastic anemia from hypocellular MDS. Both morphologic study and cytogenetic analysis are needed to help in this regard. Histologic findings such as hypogranular myeloid cells and dyserythropoiesis can be seen in aplastic anemia as well as MDS, and need to be considered along with other clinical findings when trying to differentiate these disorders. The finding of a clonal cytogenetic abnormality would be confirmatory evidence of MDS.

References

Hematology (Am Soc Hematol Educ Program), 2002:136–61.

Young NS. Acquired aplastic anemia. Ann Intern Med. 2002;136:534–6.

Answer to question 60: C

Educational objective

To recognize the optimal post-remission strategy for patients with AML and the t(8;21) translocation (core-binding factor leukemia)

Critique

Patients with AML and the t(8;21) translocation have a relatively favorable prognosis. Patients with FAB M2 morphology and the t(8;21) translocation are reported to have a higher complete remission rate than patients with other cytogenetic abnormalities. In addition, it has been demonstrated that overall outcome is improved when repetitive cycles of high-dose cytarabine are administered as post-remission therapy. Induction chemotherapy is the same as other subtypes (except APL). There is no clearly established role for any kind of transplant procedure, either autologous or allogeneic, in patients with this relatively favorable subtype of AML (core-binding factor leukemias). Transplant-related mortality for allogeneic transplants does not appear justified in this setting. There is a subgroup of patients associated with the expression of the neural cell adhesion molecule CD56, which may be linked with a shorter remission duration and extramedullary disease. Standard therapy would be four cycles of consolidation chemotherapy with high-dose cytarabine.

References

Baer MR, Stewart CC, Lawrence D, et al. Expression of the neural cell adhesion molecule CD56 is associated with short remission duration and survival in acute myeloid leukemia with t(8;21)(q22;q22). Blood. 1997;90:1643–8.

Byrd JC, Dodge RK, Caroll A, et al. Patients with t(8;21)(q22;q22) and acute myeloid leukemia have superior failure-free and overall survival when repetitive cycles of high-dose cytarabine are administered. J Clin Oncol. 1999;17:3767–75.

Byrd JC, Weiss RB, Arthur DC, et al. Extramedullary leukemia adversely affects hematologic complete remission and overall survival in patients with the t(8;21)(q22;q22): results from Cancer and Leukemia Group B 8164. J Clin Oncol. 1997;15:466–75.

Answer to question 61: C

Educational objective

To prescribe CNS prophylaxis in a child with standard risk ALL

Critique

Factors associated with a higher risk of developing CNS leukemia include higher WBC at diagnosis, infant ALL, T-cell ALL, t(9;22) [Ph+ ALL] and CNS 2 or 3 status at diagnosis. However, in the absence of preventive treatment, all patients are at increased risk of CNS relapse. A randomized study has shown that intrathecal methotrexate alone is at least as effective as triple intrathecal medications for preventive treatment of patients with standard risk ALL. Similar data for higher risk ALL are not available. Irradiation is not necessary for effective preventive treatment, with the possible exception of patients who have T-cell ALL. Craniospinal irradiation (or cranial irradiation with intrathecal methotrexate) is used for patients with CNS leukemia (CNS 3) at diagnosis or those who subsequently develop a CNS relapse.

Reference

Stork LC, Sather H, Hutchison RJ, Broxson EH, Matloub Y, Yanofsky R, et al. Comparison of mercaptopurine (MP) with thioguanine (TG) and IT methotrexate (ITM) with IT 'triples' (ITT) in children with SR-ALL: results of CCG-1952. Blood. 2002;100(Part 1):156a.

Answer to question 62: B

Educational objective

To treat relapsed aggressive non-Hodgkin lymphoma

Critique

Relapsed aggressive lymphoma has a low likelihood of cure with second-line chemotherapy alone, generally <10%. Chemosensitive relapse is thus consolidated with autologous stem cell transplantation. Allogeneic transplantation may be of value for the added graft-versus-lymphoma effect, although the morbidity and mortality of the procedure are increased as compared with autologous transplant. Rituximab maintenance therapy was not beneficial following R-CHOP as initial therapy for diffuse large B-cell lymphoma in the Eastern Cooperative Oncology Group (ECOG) 4494 study. Maintenance rituximab has not been reported in the relapsed aggressive lymphoma setting, as in this case. Radioimmunotherapy is being investigated for efficacy in relapsed aggressive lymphoma but is not currently established for this indication.

Reference

Moskowitz CH, Bertino JR, Glassman JR, et al. Ifosfamide, carboplatin, and etoposide: a highly effective cytoreduction and peripheral-blood progenitor-cell mobilization regimen for transplant-eligible patients with non-Hodgkin's lymphoma. J Clin Oncol. 1999;17:3776–85.

Answer to question 63: E

Educational objective

To recognize the preference for a CMV-negative HLA-identical donor in a CMV-negative recipient

Critique

The best donor is the HLA-identical CMV-negative brother. The sister with her pregnancies would increase the chance of graft-versus-host disease (GVHD). Moreover, she is CMV-positive and could transmit CMV to the patient. CMV remains a significant cause of post-transplant morbidity. Although trying to maximize graft-versus-leukemia effect is desirable, the ability to control severe acute GVHD remains very difficult. If an HLA-matched sibling donor is available, this donor would be chosen over a mismatched family member or an unrelated matched donor. Waiting for the cord blood is unwise, both because the patient is unlikely to remain in remission long and it is unlikely that there would be sufficient cells to transplant the patient. Unrelated donors are not used unless there is no family donor available. Moreover, the time required to find and finish typing of these donors makes it unlikely that a donor could be identified before the patient relapsed.

References

Kollman C, et al. Blood. 2001;98:2043–51.

Kollman C, Howe W, Anasetti C , Antin J, Davies S, Filipovich A, et al. Donor characteristics as risk factors in recipients after transplantation of bone marrow from unrelated donors: the effect of donor age. Blood. 2001;98:2043–51.

Answer to question 64: D

Educational objective

To recognize the prognosis of pregnancy-related thrombotic thrombocytopenic purpura

Critique

There is a clear association of pregnancy with thrombotic thrombocytopenic purpura (TTP). Most patients with TTP are women, and TTP is associated with pregnancy in about one-fourth of women of childbearing age. Therefore, counseling women about the risks of future pregnancies is a common clinical issue. There is no difference between the syndromes described as TTP and hemolytic uremic syndrome (HUS), except that patients with acute renal failure may be described as having HUS. Patients with acute renal failure relapse less frequently; therefore this woman, without renal insufficiency, may be described as having TTP and may have a significant risk for relapse. Although it is often stated that TTP occurs earlier during pregnancy and HUS occurs near term or postpartum, in fact both syndromes most often occur in the peripartum time. Classic TTP caused by ADAMTS13 deficiency most often occurs at delivery or postpartum. Although some of the very rare patients with congenital TTP caused by ADAMTS13 mutations have recurrent symptoms as infants or children, there are multiple reports of women with congenital TTP whose first episodes occur near term of their first pregnancy; they may then have frequent subsequent relapses.

This patient's risk for recurrence with a subsequent pregnancy is uncertain. Although reliable data are not available, most women who have recovered from TTP have uncomplicated subsequent pregnancies and healthy children. It would be inappropriate to advise her not to become pregnant again.

Reference

Vesely SK, Li X, McMinn JR, Terrell DR, George JN. Pregnancy outcomes after recovery from thrombotic thrombocytopenic purpura–hemolytic uremic syndrome. Transfusion. 2004;44(8):1149–58.

Answer to question 65: D

Educational objective

To manage nonimmune platelet transfusion refractoriness

Critique

Failure to achieve an adequate response to platelet transfusion is termed platelet refractoriness, if it is observed repetitively. Checking the platelet count soon after transfusion, followed by periodic counts to determine if the increment is sustained, is the best assessment of platelet transfusion response. The actual increment observed depends upon the size of the patient (blood volume) and the number of platelets transfused. A formula that accounts for these variables, termed the corrected count increment (CCI), is often used to assess response, but depends on knowing the actual platelet content of the transfusion, which is not usually available. A good increment followed by a gradual decrement in platelet count over the following day or two is the normal expectation. Poor increments caused by immediate destruction of transfused platelets usually indicate immune-mediated mechanisms such as HLA alloimmunization. Decreased post-transfusion survival following a good initial increment usually indicates a nonimmune destructive mechanism. The CCI for the transfusions in this case is approximately 5250, based on an increment of 9000, assumed dose of 3.6×10^{11} platelets for the 'four-pack' ($4 \times 0.9 \times 10^{11}$ platelets/concentrate as an average content) and surface area of 2.1 m^2. This is below the usual CCI value of 10,000–20,000 seen in most successful transfusions, but still is a detectable increment. The detectable but blunted immediate post-transfusion increment, coupled with a negative HLA antibody screen, suggests a destructive process leading to poor platelet survival rather than an antibody-mediated mechanism. It has been proven that transplantation results in a need for higher doses of platelets in order to obtain adequate increments, perhaps linked to the endothelial injury caused by preparative regimens. Because the benefit of platelet transfusion is felt to be dependent on a sustained platelet increment, this pseudo-refractoriness can be overcome through higher platelet doses. While the average platelet content for an apheresis product is approximately equivalent to a pool of four or five platelet concentrates, individual apheresis products may actually have fewer platelets than a 'four-pack' which decreases their usefulness in dose escalation. The use of HLA-matched platelets in such patients has no role because there is no evidence for alloimmunization. While crossmatching may detect platelet incompatibility missed by standard HLA antibody methods, the transfusion responses here are inconsistent with an immune mechanism. Refractoriness from ABO incompatibility has been reported, but usually in hyperimmune group O recipients of group A platelets, which is not the clinical scenario described. Platelet destruction resulting from donor-derived anti-A produced by the 'passenger lymphocytes' has also been described, but would not be seen this early post-transplant.

References

Ishida A, Handa M, Wakui M, Okamoto S, Kamakura M, Ikeda Y. Clinical factors influencing post-transfusion platelet increment in patients undergoing hematopoietic progenitor cell transplantation: a prospective analysis. Transfusion. 1998;38:839–47.

Klumpp TR, Herman JH, Gaughan JP, Russo RR, Christman RA, Goldberg SL, et al. Clinical consequences of alterations in

platelet transfusion dose: a prospective, randomized, double-blind trial. Transfusion. 1999;39:674–81.
Schiffer CA, Anderson KC, Bennett CL, Bernstein S, Elting LS, Goldsmith M, et al. Platelet transfusion for patients with cancer: clinical practice guidelines of the American Society of Clinical Oncology. J Clin Oncol. 2001;19:1519–38.

Answer to question 66: D

Educational objective

To recognize and evaluate an acquired factor VIII inhibitor

Critique

The patient has active bleeding and a prolonged APTT that almost corrects in the immediate 1 : 1 mixing study, but prolongs with the 2-h incubation. This is characteristic of some factor VIII inhibitors, and a factor VIII assay should be carried out next. If abnormal, a factor VIII inhibitor study should be performed to obtain the titer of the antibody. There is no clinical indication to order platelet aggregation studies. A lupus anticoagulant might give this pattern of laboratory findings, but it is extremely rare that it causes prolongation in the mixing study after 2 h, and lupus anticoagulants do not cause bleeding problems. von Willebrand disease would not be expected to show an abnormal mixing study in the APTT, and factor XII deficiency or inhibitor does not cause bleeding (and the deficiency should correct in the 1 : 1 mix).

References

Cohen AJ, Kessler CM. Acquired inhibitors. Bailliere's Clin Haematol. 1996;9:331–54.
Pruthi RK, Nichols WL. Autoimmune factor VIII inhibitors. Curr Opin Hematol. 1999;6:314–22.

Answer to question 67: B

Educational objective

To prescribe a transfusion product in a patient with a positive direct antiglobulin test

Critique

The provision of compatible red blood cells to a patient with a positive direct and indirect antibody test is a therapeutic challenge. In a nontransfused patient, the test results indicate the presence of autoantibodies to the patient's red blood cells. The autoantibodies typically bind to common red cell antigens, especially of the Rh group, and it is often impossible to make a compatible crossmatch. In the setting of severe anemia, it is justifiable to transfuse the 'least-incompatible' ABO/Rh-matched unit of red blood cells. The resulting hemolysis is less risky to the patient than the tissue hypoxia secondary to severe anemia. The blood bank should be asked to exclude red cell alloantibodies that can be masked by the autoantibody prior to transfusion. Alternative products are without proven benefit. Washed red blood cells are depleted of plasma proteins and leukocytes but not of red cell antigens and are of no added benefit in this context. In addition, washing red blood cells is less effective than an inline transfusion filter. Gamma irradiation kills live leukocytes but they are not a risk to this patient. HLA-compatible units lack utility in patients with autoantibodies because the antibodies that cause autoimmune hemolytic anemia are directed toward the common red cell and not the HLA antigens.

Reference

Buetens OW, Ness PM. Red blood cell transfusion in autoimmune hemolytic anemia. Curr Opin Hematol. 2003;10:429–33.

Answer to question 68: C

Educational objective

To recognize potential approaches for inducing myeloid leukemia cell differentiation

Critique

AML results from a block in myeloid differentiation because of transcriptional repression of differentiation-promoting genes. Within chromosomes, most genes are maintained in an inactive state bound in chromatin, a complex of DNA with histone and nonhistone proteins that 'shield' the DNA from proteins that activate gene expression. For a gene to be expressed, this tight complex must be unwound and made accessible to regulatory proteins. Both increased histone deacetylase (HDAC) activity and increased methylation contribute to AML pathogenesis by silencing differentiation-associated genes. Abnormal recruitment of HDAC complexes is crucial to the activity of the AML-specific fusion proteins, such as PML-RARα and AML1-ETO, suggesting that modification of the chromatin structure in the target promoters of fusion proteins represents an important mechanism of leukemogenesis. There are both *in vitro* and *in vivo* data to suggest that HDAC inhibition and/or methylation inhibition are potential therapeutic approaches in AML. Clinical trials utilizing HDAC inhibitors (e.g. valproic acid) and hypomethylating agents (e.g. decitabine) are currently in progress.

The use of all-*trans* retinoic acid (ATRA) for treatment of acute promyelocytic leukemia (APL) has proven that differentiation therapy can be successfully applied in AML. The PML-RARα fusion protein functions as a dominant negative receptor over wild-type RARα, resulting in transcriptional repression. The dominant negative effect of PML-RARα is thought to result from tighter binding of corepressors N-CoR, Sin3 and HDAC relative to RARα. Pharmacologic ATRA dissociates the corepressors from PML-RARα and relieves the differentiation block in APL blasts. In addition, ATRA treatment enhances proteolytic cleavage of PML-RARα protein in APL cells.

Nearly one-third of cases of AML harbor an abnormality of the FLT-3 receptor leading to constitutive activation of the receptor. Potential therapy may include antagonism of the FLT-3 receptor. Activation of the receptor would promote proliferation, but not differentiation, of AML blasts.

References

He LZ, Tolentino T, Grayson P, Zhong S, et al. Histone deacetylase inhibitors induce remission in transgenic models of therapy-resistant acute promyelocytic leukemia. J Clin Invest. 2001;108:1321–30.

Issa JP, Garcia-Manero G, Giles FJ, Mannari R, Thomas D, Faderl S et al. Phase I study of low-dose prolonged exposure schedules of the hypomethylating agent 5-aza-2′-deoxycytidine (Decitabine) in hematopoietic malignancies. Blood. 2004;103:1635–40.

Wang J, Saunthararajah Y, Redner RL, Liu JM. Inhibitors of histone deacetylase relieve ETO-mediated repression and induce differentiation of AML1-ETO leukemia cells. Cancer Res. 1999;59:2766–9.

Warrell RP, He LZ, Richon V, Calleja E, Pandolfi PP. Therapeutic targeting of transcription in acute promyelocytic leukemia by use of an inhibitor of histone deacetylase. J Natl Cancer Inst. 1998;90:1621–5.

Answer to question 69: B

Educational objective

To manage a pediatric patient with Fanconi anemia and myelodysplastic syndrome

Critique

The patient has Fanconi anemia and myelodysplastic syndrome. Stem cell transplant from a matched (unaffected) sibling should be considered as the initial treatment choice in Fanconi anemia patients with severe bone marrow failure, myelodysplastic syndrome or acute myeloid leukemia. Because of the increased sensitivity of Fanconi cells to DNA damage-inducing agents, attenuated alkylating agent and radiation doses or alternative agents, such as fludarabine and/or antithymocyte globulin, are required for conditioning prior to stem cell transplant. These same considerations complicate chemotherapy induction for acute myeloid leukemia in the Fanconi patient. Therefore, giving systemic chemotherapy prior to stem cell transplant conditioning entails additional risks without clear evidence of increased benefit.

Reference

Guardiola P, Socie G, Pasquini R et al. Allogeneic stem cell transplantation for Fanconi anemia: severe aplastic anemia working party of the EBMT and EUFAR. European Group for Blood and Marrow Transplantation. Bone Marrow Transplant. 1998;21(Suppl.2):S24–7.

Answer to question 70: E

Educational objective

To recognize that growth factor therapy is not indicated in patients with non-neutropenic fever

Critique

Filgrastim is not indicated for the treatment of non-neutropenic fever or infection (pneumonia) as shown by several randomized controlled trials. In a systematic review, use of filgrastim appeared to be safe with no increase in the incidence of total serious adverse events or organ dysfunction. However, the use of filgrastim was not associated with improved 28-day mortality. Epoetin alfa will have little effect on improving her hematocrit in the short term. For rare patients who refuse blood products for religious or other reasons, beginning epoetin alfa early in the course of treatment may be useful. Her thrombocytopenia is likely related to sepsis; platelet transfusions in the absence of severe thrombocytopenia and bleeding are not indicated.

References

Cheng A, Stephens D, Currie B. Granulocyte colony stimulating factor (G-CSF) as an adjunct to antibiotics in the treatment of pneumonia in adults. Cochrane Database Syst Rev. 2003;4:CD004400.

Nelson S, Heyder AM, Stone J, Bergeron MG, Daugherty S, Peterson G, et al. A randomized controlled trial of filgrastim for the treatment of hospitalized patients with multilobar pneumonia. J Infect Dis. 2000;182:970–3.

Answer to question 71: (a) D, (b) C

Educational objective

To recognize the most common genotype leading to clinical hemochromatosis, and the follow-up after the development of symptomatic disease

Critique

Most individuals who are heterozygous for either the C282Y or H63D mutation do not develop clinical iron overload in the absence of other risk factors. Homozygotes for the H63D mutation also rarely develop clinical iron overload. Over 80% of Caucasian individuals diagnosed with clinical hereditary hemochromatosis are homozygous for the C282Y mutation. In some series, 20–30% of Caucasians have no underlying genetic defect that can be identified (wild-type/wild-type).

Once cirrhosis has been documented, life expectancy even with phlebotomy will likely be shortened. Ferritin values can be expected to decrease by approximately 30 ng/mL with each unit of blood phlebotomized. Therefore it would take many months for ferritin to normalize with weekly phlebotomy. With iron unloading, malaise may improve but not the risk for hepatoma, as cirrhosis has already developed. Lifelong cancer screening with serum alfa-fetoprotein (AFP) levels and liver ultrasound is therefore recommended. Iron chelation is an inefficient method of removing iron and would be contraindicated in this patient who has a history of high frequency hearing loss.

References

Barton JC, McDonnell SM, Adams PC, Brissot P, Powell LW, Edwards CQ, et al. Management of hemochromatosis. Hemochromatosis Manage Working Group. Ann Intern Med. 1998;129:932–9.

Brandhagen DJ, Fairbanks VF, Batts KP, Thibodeau SN. Update on hereditary hemochromatosis and the *HFE* gene. Mayo Clin Proc. 1999;74:917–21.

Felitti VJ, Beutler E. New developments in hereditary hemochromatosis. Am J Med Sci. 1999;318:257–68.

Answer to question 72: A

Educational objective

To identify mitochondrial ferritin as a marker for sideroblastic anemia

Critique

The patient described has X-linked sideroblastic anemia characterized by mutations in the ALA-synthase gene. Most of the iron in the siderosome in patients with sideroblastic anemia is contained in mitochondrial ferritin and increased mitochondrial ferritin is a specific marker for sideroblastic anemia. The anemia in sideroblastic anemia is caused by disrupted erythropoiesis. Patients with sideroblastic anemia have elevated tissue iron from disordered erythropoiesis characterized by elevated serum ferritin levels. Because iron is incorporated into mitochondrial ferritin, serum iron levels are low, free erythrocyte protoporphyrin levels are high and soluble transferrin levels are high.

References

Cazzola M, Invernizzi R, Bergamaschi G, Levi S, Corsi B, Travaglino E, et al. Mitochondrial ferritin expression in erythroid cells from patients with sideroblastic anemia. Blood. 2003;101:1996–2000.

Drysdale J, Arosio P, Invernizzi R, Cazzola M, Volz A, Corsi B, et al. Mitochondrial ferritin: a new player in iron metabolism. Blood Cells Mol Dis. 2002;29:376–83.

Answer to question 73: C

Educational objective

To manage an uncomplicated sickle cell pain crisis

Critique

This patient presents with an uncomplicated pain crisis without evidence of infection, acute chest syndrome or multiorgan failure. His shallow inspiration, likely resulting from rib pain, has led to atelectasis. Aggressive incentive spirometry should be initiated to reduce the risk of acute chest syndrome. Hypotonic fluid (e.g. D5$^1/_2$ NS) should be given at a maintenance rate to avoid volume overload as this patient has no evidence of dehydration. Although adequate analgesia is imperative, meperidine should be avoided because of the short duration of action and seizure potential. Morphine or hydromorphone typically administered by patient-controlled analgesia (PCA) is preferred. There is no indication for red cell transfusion or empirical antibiotic therapy in an otherwise uncomplicated sickle cell pain crisis.

References

Bellet P, Kalinyak K, Shukla R, et al. Incentive spirometry to prevent acute pulmonary complications in sickle cell disease. N Engl J Med. 1995;333:699–703.

Benjamin LJ, Dampier CD, Jacox AK, Odesina V, Phoenix D, Shapiro B, et al. Guideline for the Management of Acute and Chronic Pain in Sickle-Cell Disease. APS Clinical Practice Guidelines Series 1. Glenview, IL: American Pain Society, 1999.

Rees DC, Olujohungbe AD, Parker NE, Stephens AD, Telfer P, Wright J. British Committee for Standards in Haematology

General Haematology Task Force by the Sickle Cell Working Party. Guidelines for the management of the acute painful crisis in sickle cell disease. Br J Haematol. 2003;120:744–52.
Steinberg MH. Management of sickle cell disease. N Engl J Med. 1999;340:1021–30.

Answer to question 74: D

Educational objective

To recognize the clinical presentation and immunohistopathologic features of systemic mastocytosis

Critique

The patient has clinical features and marrow biopsy findings suggestive of systemic mastocytosis. Clinical features include pigmented macular skin lesions, suspicious for urticaria pigmentosa, together with gastrointestinal symptoms and dermatographism attributable to histamine overproduction. A biopsy of the pigmented skin lesions would be expected to reveal infiltration of the dermis with atypical mast cells. Systemic mastocytosis is diagnosed by identifying extracutaneous tissue mast cell infiltration (in the presence or absence of associated skin lesions). Because the marrow is the most commonly involved extracutaneous tissue, aspiration and biopsy, with special stains for tryptase, CD2 and CD25 expression, usually confirm the diagnosis. The clinical signs and symptoms of systemic mastocytosis may be subtle and nonspecific. Therefore, it is important to remember this disorder in the differential diagnosis of patients with unexplained cytopenias so that the appropriate immunohistochemical stains are applied and abnormal marrow mast cell infiltration can be identified. Marrow aggregates of spindle-shaped mast cells must be differentiated from other infiltrative processes, such as non-Hodgkin lymphoma, Hodgkin lymphoma, granulomata resulting from infections or inflammatory disorders, fibrosis and tumor. Adjunctive diagnostic criteria for systemic mastocytosis include detection of the Asp-816-Val mutation of the c-*kit* gene (found in a majority of patients) and elevation of the serum tryptase level (of note, normal serum levels are found with mast cell disease confined to the skin). The mild cytopenias in this patient do not reach the criteria for 'aggressive' systemic mastocytosis; therefore, he can be managed with symptomatic and supportive treatment, but should be closely monitored.

References

Valent P, Akin C, Sperr WR, Horny HP, Arock M, Lechner K, et al. Diagnosis and treatment of systemic mastocytosis: state of the art. Br J Haematol. 2003;122:695–717.
Yavuz AS, Lipsky PE, Yavuz S, Metcalfe DD, Akin C. Evidence for the involvement of a hematopoietic progenitor cell in systemic mastocytosis from single-cell analysis of mutations in the c-*kit* gene. Blood. 2002;100:661–5.

Answer to question 75: B

Educational objective

To treat essential thrombocythemia in a pregnant patient

Critique

Women with essential thrombocythemia (ET) have a 30–40% chance of early spontaneous miscarriage. This risk does not correlate with aspirin usage or platelet count. Because this patient has suffered a prior arterial thrombotic complication, she will require ongoing therapy to control the platelet count and minimize the risk of recurrent thromboemboli. Although aspirin may not affect her risk of early miscarriage, it is a good antithrombotic choice with her history of a prior arterial event. Low-molecular-weight heparin would be a safe and appropriate agent in the setting of a recent arterial or venous event, or for secondary prophylaxis after a prior venous or obstetric event when the platelet count was in the normal range. However, the benefit of heparin in this case would likely not add to aspirin, nor would it clearly outweigh the risk of bleeding. During pregnancy, interferon-α is the platelet-lowering agent of choice, as hydroxyurea and anagrelide are potentially teratogenic. However, this patient's history of depression is a strong contraindication to interferon-α. Plateletpheresis is the best alternative method to control the platelet count. A central venous catheter should be placed for access, and the procedure will likely be required two or three times weekly throughout pregnancy and for 6 weeks' postpartum to keep the platelet count at or near the normal range.

References

Harrison CN, Green AR. Essential thrombocythemia. Hematol Oncol Clin North Am. 2003;17:1175–90.
Wright CA, Tefferi A. A single institutional experience with 43 pregnancies in essential thrombocythemia. Eur J Haematol. 2001;66:152–9.

Answer to question 76: C

Educational objective

To understand risk-adapted treatment approaches of MDS in the elderly

Critique

Patients with MDS tend to be older, have more comorbid medical conditions and are generally less able to tolerate intensive therapy of their disease. Although allogeneic transplantation is the only known curative therapy for MDS, the majority of patients diagnosed with MDS are not able to undergo such a procedure because of the unavailability of a suitable donor or their inability to tolerate intensive therapy. It is for this reason that many patients will either be treated with growth factors, such as erythropoietin or filgrastim, or may just receive supportive care with transfusions and antibiotics as needed. It would be reasonable to start this patient on growth factor therapy in an effort to decrease or eliminate transfusion requirements. If this therapy fails, supportive care with blood products would then be considered. Many biologic agents presently under study such as thalidomide and arsenic trioxide may offer potential clinical benefit without subjecting the patient to undue risk as can be seen with intensive chemotherapeutic approaches. In this situation, however, thalidomide would be relatively contraindicated given the risk of peripheral neuropathy and the pre-existing diabetes. Proceeding directly to induction chemotherapy in patients with MDS and a borderline performance status may be excessively toxic for these patients, and therefore be less likely to provide clinical benefit.

Reference

Heaney ML, Golde DW. Myelodysplasia. N Engl J Med. 1999;340:1649–60.

Answer to question 77: A

Educational objective

To recognize the optimal induction chemotherapy regimen for older adults with AML

Critique

Older adults who present with AML represent a difficult problem. Many such patients are not suitable for chemotherapy. The complete remission rate is lower for older adults, and overall survival is quite poor. There is no evidence that altering a standard induction program is beneficial. The reason for the significantly worse outcome in older adults relates to more unfavorable prognostic factors including abnormal cytogenetics, expression of multidrug resistance markers and morphology that suggests antecedent myelodysplasia. There is no evidence that giving additional agents other than daunorubicin and cytarabine is beneficial. Furthermore, there is no evidence that adding the immunoconjugate gemtuzumab ozogamicin to a standard induction regimen of daunorubicin and cytarabine is helpful.

References

Leith CP, Kopecky KL, Godwin J, et al. Acute myeloid leukemia in the elderly: assessment of multidrug resistance (MDR 1) and cytogenetics distinguishes biologic subtypes with remarkably distinct responses to standard chemotherapy. A Southwest Oncology Group Study. Blood. 1997;89:3323–9.

Lowenberg B, Zittoun R, Kerkhofs H, et al. On the value of intensive remission induction chemotherapy in elderly patients of 65+ years with acute myeloid leukemia: a randomized phase III study of the European Organization for Research and Treatment of Cancer Leukemia Group. J Clin Oncol. 1989;7:1268–74.

Rowe JM. Treatment of acute myelogenous leukemia in older adults. Leukemia. 2000;14:480–7.

Answer to question 78: B

Educational objective

To treat childhood B-cell leukemia

Critique

The clinical and laboratory findings in this patient are consistent with a diagnosis of mature B-cell acute leukemia (Burkitt leukemia). B-cell leukemia formerly carried a poor prognosis when treated with standard chemotherapy for childhood ALL. However, this disease can be cured in 80–85% of cases with 3–8 months of chemotherapy that includes cyclophosphamide, doxorubicin, dexamethasone, vincristine, high-dose methotrexate and high-dose cytosine arabinoside. Intrathecal injections of cytosine arabinoside or methotrexate are used to decrease the risk of CNS relapse. There is no evidence that more prolonged treatment improves event-free survival. Given the high cure rate with this approach, bone marrow transplantation should be reserved for patients who relapse.

Reference

Patte C, Auperin A, Michon J, Behrendt H, Leverger G, Behrendt H, et al. The Societe Française d'Oncologie Pediatrique LMB 89 protocol: highly effective multiagent chemotherapy tailored to the tumor burden and initial response in 561 unselected children with B-cell lymphomas and L3 leukemia. Blood. 2001;97:3370–9.

Answer to question 79: D

Educational objective

To treat post-transplant lymphoproliferative disorder

Critique

Post-transplant lymphoproliferative disorder (PTLD) occurs in approximately 2–5% of organ transplant patients. A minority will regress with reduction of immunosuppression; combination chemotherapy provides clinical responses but is often poorly tolerated. Recent small series have shown approximately 50% response rates in PTLD with the use of rituximab, often in conjunction with reduced immunosuppression. While the durability of response to rituximab is as yet incompletely defined, it is a reasonable approach in this setting before consideration of graft removal or chemotherapy. Some PTLDs are EBV related, usually those that arise within the first 6 months of transplantation, but response to antiviral therapy is inconsistent.

Reference

Milpied N, Vasseur B, Parquet N, Garnier JL, Antoine C, Quartier P, et al. Humanized anti-CD20 monoclonal antibody (rituximab) in post-transplant B-lymphoproliferative disorder: a retrospective analysis on 32 patients. Ann Oncol. 2000;11(Suppl.1):S113–6.

Answer to question 80: D

Educational objective

To recognize the clinical triad of veno-occlusive disease: tender hepatomegaly, ascites and >10% weight gain

Critique

The patient likely has VOD. His symptoms, his heavy treatment just prior to the transplant, liver dysfunction at the time of transplant and sonogram are all classic for the disease. The patient has not engrafted, hence liver GVHD and hematopoiesis in the liver are not possible. Moreover, GVHD does not cause tender hepatomegaly. Viral hepatitis would be unlikely to present with these symptoms or ultrasound findings. Likewise, a fatty liver from hyperalimentation would be unlikely in 2 days.

Reference

Arai S, Lee LA, Vogelsang GB. A systematic approach to hepatic complications in hematopoietic stem cell transplantation. J Hematother Stem Cell Res. 2002;11:215–30.

Answer to question 81: A

Educational objective

To manage pre-eclampsia

Critique

Although the onset of pre-eclampsia is typically prior to delivery with recovery following delivery, pre-eclampsia can begin following delivery, as in this woman. Pre-eclampsia is most common during or following a woman's first pregnancy, and it may be more common in African-American than in Caucasian women. The key diagnostic feature in this woman is the onset of severe hypertension. The visual abnormality is characteristic of pre-eclampsia; thrombocytopenia and microangiopathic hemolysis commonly occur in severe pre-eclampsia and the onset of thrombocytopenia can be this sudden and severe. The abnormal liver function tests suggest the obstetric complication associated with pre-eclampsia described as HELLP (*h*emolysis, *e*levated *l*iver function tests, *l*ow *p*latelets) syndrome.

This patient can be safely observed with no treatment intervention. Spontaneous recovery should be prompt; a clear response documented within the next 2 days confirms the diagnosis of pre-eclampsia. Some reports have described plasma exchange for severe pre-eclampsia or HELLP syndrome, but this woman's illness is not severe enough to justify the risks of plasma exchange. The presence of severe hypertension diminishes the possibility of TTP. Although sepsis is always a concern at or soon after delivery, and systemic lupus erythematosus may cause these abnormalities, these diagnoses are much less likely.

Reference

McMinn JR, George JN. Evaluation of women with clinically suspected thrombotic thrombocytopenic purpura–hemolytic uremic syndrome during pregnancy. J Clin Apheresis. 2001;16:202–9.

Answer to question 82: A

Educational objective

To treat thrombotic thrombocytopenic purpura

Critique

This is an example of thrombotic thrombocytopenic purpura (TTP) with four of the five symptoms or signs needed for the diagnosis (fever, neurologic symptoms, thrombocytopenia, microangiopathic hemolysis, renal failure). Sometimes, the clinical manifestation of TTP seems identical to hemolytic uremic syndrome because TTP can cause renal impairment, but this patient has no manifestations of kidney dysfunction. TTP has been linked to perturbations in the ADAMTS13 metalloprotease that affect the enzymatic cleavage of von Willebrand (VW) multimers. An imbalance in circulating very large VW multimers ensues, causing primary platelet activation and microangiopathy. TTP has been shown to respond to infusion of plasma products such as FFP, which replaces the enzyme and normalizes the balance of VW multimers. Numerous series and one randomized study in TTP have demonstrated significantly better response to daily plasma exchange through apheresis rather than simple plasma infusion. Presumably, this is because of the much larger amount of plasma that can be infused during exchange without causing volume overload. Occasionally, the supernatant from cryoprecipitate production is used, which is devoid of most VW, and but does contain the protease. Because the thrombocytopenia in TTP is a destructive process, platelet transfusion causes only a transient increment at best. Also, worsening of TTP, sometimes leading to fatality, has been reported directly following platelet transfusion, and so transfusion should be reserved for life-threatening hemorrhage in view of the risks. While steroids can be used to reduce the autoantibodies, and at least one study has suggested a survival advantage for TTP patients given steroids, their use is adjunctive to the prompt initiation of plasma exchange. Many immune-mediated thrombocytopenias have been shown to respond to intravenous immunoglobulin (IVIG), and the immune modulation attributed to IVIG may also aid in reducing the autoantibody. However, effectiveness of IVIG in the initial therapy of TTP has not been demonstrated, and daily plasma exchange would remove much of the transfused IVIG, making its use impractical.

References

Koo AP. Overview of therapeutic apheresis in the USA. Ther Apher. 1999;3:4–7.

McLeod BC. Introduction to the third special issue: clinical applications of therapeutic apheresis. J Clin Apher. 2000;15:1–5.

Moake JL. Thrombotic microangiopathies. N Engl J Med. 2002;347:589–600.

Answer to question 83: C

Educational objective

To evaluate a patient with low levels of factor VIII

Critique

The patient has a lifelong history of bleeding, a positive family history of bleeding and her factor VIII level is low. Her VWF levels are normal and her bleeding has occurred after invasive procedures (not necessarily mucosal bleeding), making type 1, type 3, or type 2A, 2B or 2M von Willebrand disease (VWD) unlikely. Although she could be a carrier for hemophilia A with extreme lyonization, the only other family bleeding history is in a female, making this unlikely. The more likely diagnosis is type 2N VWD, and a binding assay using her VWF to assess its ability to bind factor VIII would be definitive. The RIPA and VWF multimer studies are expected to be normal, and the platelet aggregations and lupus anticoagulant assay would not be indicated with this isolated factor VIII deficiency.

References

Mazurier C, Goudemand J, Hilbert L, Caron C, Fressinaud E, Meyer D. Type 2N von Willebrand disease: clinical manifestations, pathophysiology, laboratory diagnosis and molecular biology. Best Pract Res Clin Haematol. 2001;14:337–47.

Rick ME, Williams SB, Sacher RA, McKeown LP. Thrombocytopenia associated with pregnancy in a patient with type IIb von Willebrand's disease. Blood. 1987;69:786–9.

Answer to question 84: A

Educational objective

To manage postoperative bleeding

Critique

Postoperative bleeding after CABG has several possible causes. Thrombocytopenia and an acquired secretion defect arise from activation by the bypass pump and hypothermia. Coagulation proteins may also be affected. A previously unrecognized hemostatic defect could also be unmasked. Bleeding due to these causes is usually delayed and slow, unlike this patient's bleeding which is immediate and brisk. The most common cause of immediate brisk postoperative bleeding is a bleeding vessel in the operative field. The absence of other evidence of a systemic bleeding disorder confirms the impression that surgical bleeding is the most significant risk. Although infusion of the proposed hemostatic agents or platelets might have a beneficial effect on bleeding in this patient, surgery should not be delayed.

Reference

Lind SE, Marks PW, Ewenstein BM. Hemostatic system. In: Handin RI, Lux SE, Stossel TP, eds. Blood, Principles and Practice of Hematology. Philadelphia: Lippincott Williams & Wilkins, 2002:959.

Answer to question 85: B

Educational objective

To recognize the use of DNA microarray studies

Critique

DNA microarrays are a relatively new technology developed to evaluate whole genome patterns of expression. The starting material for such studies is RNA, as 'gene expression' refers to levels of messenger RNA (mRNA). DNA microarrays do not evaluate protein levels. In fact, this is a limitation of the technology; it does not assess global changes in protein level or post-translational modifications.

The DNA microarray is still a research tool. Although microarray technology has generated interesting hypotheses that may ultimately affect clinical care, it is not yet a validated tool for diagnosis or for clinical management.

Reference

Russo G, Zegar C, Giordano A. Advantages and limitations of microarray technology in human cancer [Review]. Oncogene. 2003;22:6497–507.

Answer to question 86: C

Educational objective

To diagnose and appropriately manage drug-induced aplastic anemia in an elderly patient

Critique

Aplastic anemia can be triggered by medications. Clopidogrel has a reported association with aplastic anemia, although it is a very rare complication (a more frequent association was with ticlopidine, an antiplatelet agent that preceded clopidogrel). Other medications associated with aplastic anemia include chloramphenicol, phenylbutazone, indometacin, diclofenac sodium and gold. Of patients with aplastic anemia, 10–20% have spontaneous improvement of their blood counts within 2–4 weeks of presentation. Spontaneous remission is more common if there is an identified etiology such as a medication or infection. Drug-induced aplastic anemia can be successfully treated with immunosuppression. Because of her advanced age, if there is no response to discontinuation of clopidogrel within 14–21 days, immunosuppression will provide the best chance of recovery.

Although aspirin is not a cause of aplastic anemia, it should be stopped in a patient with severe thrombocytopenia. The other medications are necessary to treat her other underlying medical conditions, and are unlikely to have caused her aplastic anemia. Therefore, they should not be discontinued.

References

Lee JH, Lee JH, Shin YR et al. Spontaneous remission of aplastic anemia: a retrospective analysis. Haematologica. 2001;86:928–33.

Love BB, Biller J, Gent M. Adverse hematological effects of ticlopidine: prevention, recognition and management. Drug Saf. 1998;19:89–98.

Answer to question 87: B

Educational objective

To recognize a rare, serious complication of filgrastim

Critique

The most likely diagnosis is splenic rupture, a rare complication of filgrastim described in both normal donors and patients with hematologic malignancies. Filgrastim has been shown to increase splenic size frequently in normal stem cell donors. In almost all cases the enlargement has been asymptomatic and with no clinical consequences. The rapid decline in his hematocrit without evidence for gastrointestinal bleeding or hemolysis supports a diagnosis of intra-abdominal blood loss. Infectious causes for his abdominal pain in the absence of fever would be less likely. Filgrastim occasionally produces mild to moderate bone pain. Serum sickness has not been described from treatment with either filgrastim or epoetin alfa.

References

Becker PS, Wagle M, Matous S, Swanson RS, Pihan G, Lowry PA, et al. Spontaneous splenic rupture following administration of granulocyte colony-stimulating factor (G–CSF): occurrence in an allogeneic donor of peripheral blood stem cells. Biol Blood Marrow Transplant. 1997;3:45–9.

Stroncek D, Shawker T, Follmann D, Leitman SF. G-CSF-induced spleen size changes in peripheral blood progenitor cell donors. Transfusion. 2003;43:609–13.

Answer to question 88: D

Educational objective

To understand the interpretation and subsequent implications of genetic test results in hereditary hemochromatosis

Critique

Patients often present to the hematologist for interpretation of genetic screening for hemochromatosis. The hematologist must therefore be comfortable in both the interpretation and prognostic implications of these findings. This patient's genotype is H63D/wild-type, which is only rarely associated with clinical hemochromatosis in the absence of other risk factors for iron overload such as hepatitis C or excessive alcohol intake. The patient will therefore not likely develop iron overload later in life. He has a 50% risk of passing on the H63D mutation to his children. Phlebotomy is not recommended unless iron overload is documented. The genotype H63D/wild-type is not rare, occurring in 20–24% of the Caucasian population.

References

Barton JC, McDonnell SM, Adams PC, Brissot P, Powell LW, Edwards CQ, et al. Management of hemochromatosis. Hemochromatosis Manage Working Group. Ann Intern Med. 1998;129:932–9.

Bomford A. Genetics of haemochromatosis. Lancet. 2002;360:1673–81.

Brandhagen DJ, Fairbanks VF, Batts KP, Thibodeau SN. Update on hereditary hemochromatosis and the *HFE* gene. Mayo Clin Proc. 1999;74:917–21.

Hanson EH, Imperatore G, Burke W. *HFE* gene and hereditary hemochromatosis: a HuGE review. Human Genome Epidemiology. Am J Epidemiol. 2001;154:193–206.

Answer to question 89: C

Educational objective

To recognize the erythrocyte abnormality responsible for type 1 congenital dyserythropoietic anemia (CDA)

Critique

The CDAs are a group of disorders characterized by anemia, multinucleated erythroid precursors in the marrow, ineffective erythropoiesis and iron excess. Type 1 CDA has characteristic erythroid features in the marrow as described in this case. Type 1 CDA has recently been linked to an abnormality in codanin-1, a protein with no obvious transmembrane domain which may be involved in nuclear envelope integrity, conceivably related to microtubule attachments. Type 1 CDA is not associated with disorders of ankyrin, spectrin, membrane glycoproteins or Na^+/K^+ ATPase. No effective treatment is available for type 1 CDA, and most patients do not require transfusion, which is fortunate because dyserythropoiesis leads to iron overload in later life.

Reference

Dgany O, Avidan N, Delaunay J, et al. Congenital dyserythropoietic anemia type I is caused by mutations in codanin-1. Am J Hum Genet. 2002;71:1467–74.

Answer to question 90: A

Educational objective

To recognize the risks of hydroxyurea therapy

Critique

Hydroxyurea is the only disease-modifying medication currently FDA-approved for the management of sickle cell disease. This agent is considered teratogenic, and so effective birth control needs to be practiced concurrently. In a controlled randomized clinical trial, hydroxyurea has been shown to decrease the incidence of painful episodes, acute chest syndrome and transfusion requirements in hemoglobin SS patients. Excessive leukemia risk has not been definitively demonstrated in patients with sickle cell disease but the risk continues to be debated in the treatment of myeloproliferative disorders. Because of continued uncertainty of leukemic risk, this issue should be discussed with the patient prior to prescribing the drug. Hydroxyurea is thought to be useful for treating patients with moderate to severe symptoms, both in adults as well as children with hemoglobin SS disease. Because of her frequent admissions for painful episodes, initiation of hydroxyurea would be appropriate.

References

Amrolia PJ, Almeida A, Davies SC, Roberts IA. Therapeutic challenges in childhood sickle cell disease. II. A problem-orientated approach. *Br J Haematol.* 2003;120:737–43.

Amrolia PJ, Almeida A, Halsey C, Roberts IA, Davies SC. Therapeutic challenges in childhood sickle cell disease. I. Current and future treatment options. *Br J Haematol.* 2003;120:725–36.

Charache S, Terrin ML, Moore RD, Dover GJ, Barton FB, Eckert SV, et al. Effect of hydroxyurea on the frequency of painful crises in sickle cell anemia. Investigators of the Multicenter Study of Hydroxyurea in Sickle Cell Anemia. N Engl J Med. 1995;332:1317–22.

Steinberg MH, Barton F, Castro O, Pegelow CH, Ballas SK, Kutlar A, et al. Effect of hydroxyurea on mortality and morbidity in adult sickle cell anemia: risks and benefits up to 9 years of treatment. JAMA. 2003; 289:1645–51.

Answer to question 91: C

Educational objective

To recognize the appropriate medical management of severe congenital neutropenia

Critique

This child has clinical and laboratory features that strongly support a diagnosis of severe congenital neutropenia (SCN). Many patients with SCN require a filgrastim dosage in excess of 5 μg/kg/day to achieve a neutrophil count of ≥1000/μL. The dosage should be increased every 3–5 days until a response is obtained. Patients with SCN should continue to receive filgrastim to maintain the neutrophil count in the range of 1000–1500/μL. Some experts recommend empirically increasing this dosage in children who are febrile or have other signs that suggest an infection. The risk of transformation to MDS or AML is estimated to be 10–15% in patients with SCN. Although stem cell transplantation is a reasonable consideration in children with SCN who have an HLA-matched sibling donor, transplants from unrelated donors are not recommended unless the patient is refractory to filgrastim. Approximately 15% of patients with SCN do not respond to filgrastim.

References

Banerjee A, Shannon KM. Leukemic transformation in patients with severe congenital neutropenia. J Pediatr Hematol Oncol. 2001;23:487–95.

Dale DC, Bonilla MA, Davis MW et al. A randomized controlled phase III trial of recombinant human granulocyte colony-stimulating factor (filgrastim) for treatment of severe chronic neutropenia. Blood. 1993;81:2496–502.

Answer to question 92: C

Educational objective

To recognize the mechanisms of bleeding complications with essential thrombocythemia

Critique

The prolonged activated partial thromboplastin time (APTT) in this patient and correction by a 1 : 1 mixture with normal plasma indicate coagulation factor deficiency. The correction with a 1 : 1 mix also excludes an acquired coagulation inhibitor, such as a lupus anticoagulant or factor VIII inhibitor. Neither lupus anticoagulant activity nor a factor VIII inhibitor are causally associated with underlying essential thrombocythemia (ET). If lupus anticoagulant activity was detected, it might increase further the patient's risk of a thromboembolic complication, but would not explain bleeding. If a factor VIII inhibitor was detected, it could explain the bleeding diathesis but should also prompt an evaluation for an occult malignancy or other etiologic trigger. The prolonged APTT in this case most likely reflects an acquired deficiency of von Willebrand factor (VWF). Acquired VWF deficiency is associated with extreme thrombocytosis in ET and other myeloproliferative disorders because the platelets bind to and clear large VWF multimers, leading to an acquired type 2 von Willebrand disease (VWD). The acquired type 2 VWD has been described in patients with platelet counts in the range of 1,000,000–2,000,000/μL, and is corrected by normalizing the platelet count. Because this patient has no active bleeding and is clinically stable, hydroxyurea would be a satisfactory initial cytoreductive treatment. Plateletpheresis should be carried out to reduce the platelet count rapidly if the patient is bleeding or unstable.

References

Tefferi A. Recent progress in the pathogenesis and management of essential thrombocythemia. Leuk Res. 2001;25:369–77.

Van Genderen PJ, Leenknegt H, Michiels JJ, Budde U. Acquired von Willebrand disease in myeloproliferative disorders. Leuk Lymphoma. 1996;22(Suppl.1):79–82.

Answer to question 93: C

Educational objective

To recognize the effects of 5-azacitidine in patients with MDS

Critique

5-Azacitidine (azacitidine) and 5-aza-2′-deoxycitidine (decitabine) are agents presently undergoing study that may induce a response via their hypomethylating properties. Both agents have shown promise in improving transfusion requirements and delaying progression to AML in patients with MDS. Although 5-azacitidine did not produce a large number of complete responses (CR), Silverman et al. reported that 5-azacitidine induced a response in 60% of patients (7% CR, 16% partial response and 37% with hematologic improvement) and improved the time to progression to AML or death when compared with supportive care. When used in higher doses, myelosuppression has been quite commonly seen with 5-azacitidine. This effect is not restricted to myeloblasts, and is not thought to be a consequence of the hypomethylating properties.

Reference

Silverman LR, Demakos EP, Peterson BL, Kornblith AB, Holland JC, Odchimar-Reissig R, et al. Randomized controlled trial of azacitidine in patients with the myelodysplastic syndrome: a study of the cancer and leukaemia group B. J Clin Oncol. 2002;20:2429–40.

Answer to question 94: C

Educational objective
To recognize the features of AML with the t(16;16) translocation

Critique
Acute myeloid leukemia FAB M4 with the t(16;16) translocation is associated with fusion of the *MHY11* and *CBFβ* genes. It is one of the core-binding factor leukemias. Such patients often have an abundance of abnormal eosinophils. These patients have a relatively favorable prognosis. Induction therapy, as with other subtypes of AML (except APL), includes daunorubicin plus cytarabine. In general, consolidation chemotherapy includes 2–4 courses of high-dose cytarabine. The benefits of stem cell transplantation in first remission have not been established.

References
Costello R, Sainty D, Lecine P, et al. Detection of *CBFβ-MYH11* fusion transcripts in acute myeloid leukemia: heterogeneity of cytological and molecular characteristics. Leukemia. 1997;11:644–50.

Delaunay J, Vey N, Leblanc T, et al. Prognosis of inv(16)/t(16;16) acute myeloid leukemia (AML): a survey of 110 cases from the French AML Intergroup. Blood. 2003;102:462–9.

Answer to question 95: B

Educational objective
To identify treatment of adult T-cell lymphoblastic lymphoma

Critique
T-lymphoblastic lymphoma (precursor T-lymphoblastic leukemia/lymphoma) is most commonly seen in adolescent males, frequently with an anterior mediastinal mass and in almost all cases with peripheral blood and marrow involvement. Approximately 8% of patients have positive spinal fluid cytology at diagnosis. Intrathecal CNS prophylaxis is indicated in all patients, because the CNS relapse rate is over 30% in those patients not receiving this therapy. The risk is somewhat higher for patients with T-cell lineage or mature B-cell lineage as compared with precursor B-cell phenotypes, and also higher for patients with hyperleukocytosis of circulating blasts. Systemic high-dose chemotherapy may decrease the risk of CNS recurrence but is not sufficient to preclude intrathecal therapy. An aggressive multiagent chemotherapy regimen like that used in ALL is indicated for lymphoblastic lymphoma. CHOP chemotherapy with or without radiation would be appropriate for large cell lymphoma of the mediastinum, but would not be adequate for lymphoblastic lymphoma. Stem cell transplantation is being investigated for high-risk patients in first remission, but would not be employed prior to induction chemotherapy.

References
Le Gouill S, Lepretre S, Briere J, Morel P, Bouabdallah R, Raffoux E, et al. Adult lymphoblastic lymphoma: a retrospective analysis of 92 patients under 61 years included in the LNH87/93 trials. Leukemia. 2003;17:2220–4.

Thomas DA, Kantarjian HM. Lymphoblastic lymphoma. Hematol Oncol Clin North Am. 2001;15:51.

Answer to question 96: A

Educational objective
Management of a patient with MALT lymphoma

Critique
Extranodal marginal zone B-cell lymphomas of MALT type are indolent and typically have a long natural history. They often present as stage IE disease involving the stomach, gastrointestinal tract, salivary glands, lung, soft tissue or periorbital sites. There is no established survival benefit for radiotherapy or systemic therapy in patients with fully resected or asymptomatic residual disease, and in this case watchful waiting with periodic examination and imaging studies is appropriate. Unlike most other subtypes of NHL, PET scans are frequently negative in MALT lymphoma and in this case would not change management even if otherwise occult disease was found.

Reference
Cavalli F, Isaacson PG, Gascoyne RD, Zucca E. MALT lymphomas. Hematology. 2001;241–58.

Answer to question 97: E

Educational objective
To evaluate a patient with post-transplant diarrhea

Critique
This patient most likely has acute GVHD, brought on by low to absent cyclosporine resulting from a preceding viral illness. It is also possible that the patient now has a secondary opportunistic infection, CMV enteritis or other

viral illness. To evaluate this, all of the studies listed are indicated except chimerism studies. There is no indication that the patient is losing his graft and chimerism studies will not help differentiate between GVHD and infection.

Reference

Vogelsang GB, Lee L, Bensen-Kennedy DM. Pathogenesis and treatment of graft-versus-host disease after bone marrow transplant. Ann Rev Med. 2002;54:29–52.

Answer to question 98: B

Educational objective

To recognize that systemic metastatic carcinoma can mimic thrombotic thrombocytopenic purpura (TTP)

Critique

The important abnormality in this woman is her large breast mass. This is most likely carcinoma, and systemic metastatic breast carcinoma can cause all of her abnormalities: pulmonary micrometastases mimicking thromboemboli, and marrow metastases causing the leukoerythroblastic reaction. A bone marrow biopsy should confirm the diagnosis of systemic metastatic carcinoma; a normal bone marrow aspirate and biopsy would exclude this diagnosis.

Systemic metastatic carcinoma can cause all features of TTP. DIC may not be present with metastatic carcinoma. Even at autopsy, metastatic carcinoma can mimic TTP with the presence of tumor thrombi in small vessels of all organs. The thrombi are composed of tumor cells, but proximal to the tumor thrombi are platelet thrombi that, when first seen, suggest TTP.

In this patient, the pulmonary emboli are metastatic carcinoma; an inferior vena cava filter is not appropriate in the absence of lower extremity venous thrombosis. Megaloblastic anemia can cause many features of TTP: thrombocytopenia, anemia with severe poikilocytosis suggesting the appearance of schistocytes, evidence for hemolysis and neurologic abnormalities. However, in this woman, the high white blood cell count is not consistent with megaloblastic anemia. Myeloid metaplasia with myelofibrosis causing severe thrombocytopenia is unlikely in the absence of splenomegaly.

References

Antman KH, Skarin AT, Mayer RJ, Hargreaves HK, Canellos GP. Microangiopathic hemolytic anemia and cancer: a review. Medicine. 1979;58:377–84.

Systrom DM, Mark EJ. Case records: a 55-year-old woman with acute respiratory failure and radiographically clear lungs. N Engl J Med. 1995;332:1700–8.

Answer to question 99: C

Educational objective

To treat coagulopathy after massive transfusion

Critique

When patients receive more than one blood volume of transfused packed red cells in less than 24 h, they are considered to have had a massive transfusion. Packed red cells are devoid of viable platelets and plasma, and replacing large amounts of blood with packed cells and crystalloid fluid in a short time not only fails to replace the factors and platelets lost through hemorrhage, but also leads to dilution of remaining platelets and plasma factors. This patient has diffuse bleeding which can be attributed to the multifactorial coagulopathy caused by the massive transfusion. There is laboratory evidence of either depletion of clotting factors or disseminated intravascular coagulopathy (DIC). Further testing of the fibrinogen and D-dimer levels can help sort this out, but initial transfusion support with fresh frozen plasma (FFP) as a global replacement for lost plasma is warranted. Cryoprecipitate is a rich source of concentrated fibrinogen, but contains few other clotting factors and is used as an adjunct to FFP in this setting. While dilutional thrombocytopenia is often the first abnormality in massive transfusion, the platelet count here is above the usual number felt to be associated with bleeding and platelet concentrates would probably not be of benefit. While whole blood during a massive hemorrhage may treat hypovolemia as well as the red cell deficit, the presence of many factors may be diminished, and FFP is a better product choice because it can replace any missing factors if used in sufficient quantity. In addition, few blood centers keep whole blood in inventory because processing donor blood into the various components that can target a particular deficit is the preferred method of blood product manufacture. Further use of packed cells to maintain oxygen-carrying capacity may be warranted, but will not be useful in treating the coagulopathy.

References

Herman JH. Blood component therapy for the bleeding patient: practical issues. Am J Anesthesiol. 1998;25:121–6.

Reiss RF. Hemostatic defects in massive transfusion: rapid diagnosis and management. Am J Crit Care. 2000;9:158–65.

Answer to question 100: D

Educational objective

To diagnose lymphoplasmacytic lymphoma

Critique

Chronic lymphocytic leukemias are CD5 and CD23 positive. Multiple myeloma cells are typically negative for CD20, and positive for surface immunoglobulin, CD38 and occasionally CD10. CD5 is expressed and CD38 is negative in mantle cell lymphoma. Lymphoplasmacytic lymphomas typically express CD20, CD38 and surface immunoglobulin and do not express CD5, CD10 and CD23.

Reference

Jaffe ES, Harris NL, Stein H, Vardiman JW et al. WHO Tumours of Haematopoietic and Lymphoid Tissues. Lyon: IARC Press, 2001.

Answer to question 101: C

Educational objective

To recognize the diagnostic uses of RFLP analysis

Critique

RFLPs detect constitutional inherited variations or polymorphisms in DNA that create or abolish restriction enzyme sites. Most RFLPs are located in the noncoding region of genes. These polymorphisms are 'innocent bystanders' that are inherited with the disease-causing mutations but are not themselves pathogenic. Factor V Leiden and sickle cell disease are rare examples of single-base pathogenic mutations that may be directly detected by restriction digestion after PCR amplification of the relevant gene. Western blot analysis is used to detect protein not nucleic acid.

References

Cao A, Galanello R, Rosatelli MC. Prenatal diagnosis and screening of the haemoglobinopathies. Baillière's Clin Haematol. 1998;11:215–38.

Keeney S, Salden A, Hay C, Cumming A. A whole blood, multiplex PCR detection method for factor V Leiden and the prothrombin G20210A variant. Thromb Haemost. 1999;81:464–5.

Answer to question 102: D

Educational objective

To recognize platelet dysfunction associated with myelodysplastic syndrome

Critique

Myelodysplastic syndrome (MDS) is a clonal proliferative disorder most likely originating at the level of a pluripotent stem cell. As stem cells already have an active self-renewal program, they may be more likely to persist long enough to acquire the genetic hits required for transformation. Initially, using isozyme analysis of glucose-6-phosphate dehydrogenase (G6PD) heterozygous females, granulocytes, erythrocytes and platelets in patients with MDS were demonstrated to express a single isozyme (suggesting a clonal origin). Since then, molecular analyses of other loci, such as the androgen receptor gene on the X chromosome, have confirmed these impressions. In this patient with MDS, all three lineages are derived from the malignant clone. Even though the platelet count is seemingly adequate ($>10–50 \times 10^9$/L), platelet function may be impaired (as a consequence of descending from an abnormal stem cell). The peripheral blood smear findings are not explained by answers A–C and E.

References

Hotta T. Clonality in hematopoietic disorders. Int J Hematol. 1997;66:403.

Lichtman MA. The stem cell in the pathogenesis and treatment of myelogenous leukemia: a perspective. Leukemia. 2001;15:1489–94.

Answer to question 103: C

Educational objective

To recognize the indications for dose reduction rather than growth factor therapy for chemotherapy-induced febrile neutropenia

Critique

Filgrastim used preventatively is indicated when the risk of febrile neutropenia is ≥40%. Filgrastim shortens the absolute period of neutropenia, reduces the incidence of febrile neutropenia and reduces hospital days without improvement in mortality and disease-free survival. Although a number of randomized controlled trials are testing the efficacy of dose escalation or dose density in a variety of solid tumors, there is no evidence to date that these approaches have led to improved survival. When two or more chemotherapy regimens have equal antitumor effects and survival rates for a particular malignancy or stage of disease, a regimen that does not rely on filgrastim for support (less myelotoxic) is preferred. Dose reduction as opposed to maintaining dose is favored initially after patients develop fever and neutropenia. Regimens used in breast cancer that administer chemotherapy and filgrastim over shorter intervals ('dose dense' regimens) are currently being tested, but do not constitute standard of care.

References

Berghmans T, Paesmans M, Lafitte JJ, Mascaux C, Meert AP, Sculier JP. Role of granulocyte and granulocyte-macrophage colony-stimulating factors in the treatment of small-cell lung cancer: a systematic review of the literature with methodological assessment and meta-analysis. Lung Cancer. 2002;37:115–23.

Clark OA, Lyman G, Castro AA, Clark LG, Djulbegovic B. Colony stimulating factors for chemotherapy induced febrile neutropenia. Cochrane Database Syst Rev. 2003;3:CD003039.

Savarese D, Hsieh C, Stewart FM. Clinical impact of chemotherapy dose escalation. J Clin Oncol. 1997;15:2981–95.

Answer to question 104: D

Educational objective

To recognize the clinical presentation and laboratory evaluation in a patient with suspected acute intermittent porphyria

Critique

Despite repeated extensive evaluation for abdominal pain, no obvious etiology has been identified in this patient. This history is fairly common for acute intermittent porphyria (AIP). In addition, this patient is described as emotionally labile, on oral contraception and was well prior to puberty, all supporting the diagnosis. The proper diagnostic test is a 24-h urine study for ALA and PBG collected during an acute crisis without exposure to light. Urine uroporphyrin levels are useful in the diagnosis of porphyria cutanea tarda, not AIP. There is no cutaneous involvement in AIP so skin biopsy is unnecessary. Red cell PBG levels may identify carriers of AIP, but many individuals who harbor this mutation are asymptomatic and documentation of a carrier state would not confirm causality for the patient's clinical symptoms. It is unlikely that further gastrointestinal evaluation would be revealing.

References

Daniell WE, Stockbridge HL, Labbe RF, Woods JS, Anderson KE, Bissel DM, *et al.* Environmental chemical exposures and disturbances of heme synthesis. Environ Health Perspect. 1997;105(Suppl.1):37–53.

Gonzalez-Arriaza HL, Bostwick JM. Acute porphyrias: a case report and review. Am J Psychiatry. 2003;160:450–9.

Thadani H, Deacon A, Peters T. Diagnosis and management of porphyria. Br Med J. 2000;320:1647–51.

Answer to question 105: D

Educational objective

To recognize the association of pernicious anemia with other autoimmune disorders such as autoimmune thyroid disease leading to hypothyroidism

Critique

In cobalamin deficiency states, repletion of cobalamin in the standard doses used in this patient results in a reticulocytosis that begins within days of initiating treatment. Gradual correction of anemia occurs over a period of weeks. After 4 weeks of adequate therapy, this patient does not have an appropriate reticulocyte response and her anemia is not correcting, indicating an additional problem. Patients with pernicious anemia are at increased risk of other autoimmune disorders, including thyroiditis. Hypothyroidism can result in macrocytic anemia because of an inadequate bone marrow production state.

This problem is unlikely to be caused by iron deficiency because good iron stores are noted in the bone marrow. The occurrence of a concomitant hemolytic anemia with a high LDH or positive Coombs test would be expected to result in reticulocytosis. Abnormal liver function would not be expected to suppress erythropoiesis.

References

Carmel R, Spencer C. Clinical and subclinical thyroid disorders associated with pernicious anemia: observations on abnormal thyroid-stimulating hormone levels and on a possible association of blood group O with hyperthyroidism. Arch Intern Med. 1982;142:1465–9.

Ottesen M, Feldt-Rasmussen U, Andersen J, Hippe E, Schoube A. Thyroid function and autoimmunity in pernicious anemia before and during cyanocobalamin treatment. J Endocrinol Invest. 1995;18:91–7.

Answer to question 106: D

Educational objective

To recognize the clinical presentation of warm autoimmune hemolytic anemia and differentiate the laboratory and blood bank findings from cold agglutinin disease

Critique

This patient with known rheumatoid arthritis presents with clinical findings, laboratory abnormalities and spherocytes on the blood smear, which all suggest warm autoimmune hemolytic anemia (WAIHA). The autoantibody in this condition is usually a panreactive IgG antibody. This often makes the detection of underlying alloantibodies more difficult, and specific techniques are needed to absorb the autoantibody, thus allowing an acceptable type and screen to be performed. The test used to diagnosis autoimmune hemolytic anemia is the direct antiglobulin test (DAT, direct Coombs), which will be positive for IgG alone, or both IgG and complement. In cold agglutinin disease, which is IgM-mediated, the DAT is usually positive for complement only. With cold agglutinin disease there may be visible red cell agglutination upon review of the peripheral blood smear, which is not seen in WAIHA. In cold agglutinin disease, when the blood sample is warmed to 37°C and the peripheral blood smear is prepared promptly, red cell agglutination may be avoided. As in hereditary spherocytosis (HS), the osmotic fragility test is often abnormal in WAIHA secondary to the presence of osmotically fragile spherocytic-shaped red blood cells in both of these conditions.

References

Buetens OW, Ness PM. Red blood cell transfusion in autoimmune hemolytic anemia. Curr Opin Hematol. 2003;10:429–33.

Gehrs BC, Freidberg RC. Autoimmune hemolytic anemia. Am J Hematol. 2002;69:258–71.

Answer to question 107: B

Educational objective

To diagnose Langerhans cell histiocytosis

Critique

Langerhans cell histiocytosis (LCH) is a clonal disorder with a myriad of clinical presentations that may include isolated or multiple bone lesions and aggressive multisystem disease with visceral manifestations. In this patient, a smear of the ear discharge might show diagnostic histiocytes ($S100^+$, $CD1a^+$, Birbeck granule positive). She has clinical involvement of the skin and lymph nodes, which establishes the presence of multisystem disease. A skeletal survey, bone scan, chest radiograph, bone marrow biopsy and liver function studies should ultimately be performed to measure the extent of disease; however, a tissue biopsy to make the correct diagnosis is the most appropriate next step. Biospy of a pathologic lymph node will establish the correct diagnosis and is less invasive than curettage of the mastoid. Whereas curettage or radiation of an affected bone may be the only treatment that is required for patients in whom the disease is limited to the bone, this patient will require systemic treatment if her lymph node biopsy confirms multisystem disease. LCH frequently follows a protracted course characterized by long remissions and late relapses that are amenable to further treatment. Many cases of LCH respond to chemotherapeutic agents such as vinblastine, prednisone and etoposide, and these drugs are a mainstay of modern treatment regimens. Some patients with LCH present with (or later develop) diabetes insipidus resulting from infiltration of the posterior pituitary. The worst outcomes are in children who are diagnosed early in life with multisystem disease. Such patients frequently demonstrate brief or incomplete responses to chemotherapy. Hematopoietic stem cell transplantation may cure some high-risk patients.

References

Titgemeyer C, Grois N, Minkov M, Flucher-Wolfram B, Gatterer-Menz I, Gadner H. Pattern and course of single-system disease in Langerhans cell histiocytosis data from the DAL-HX 83- and 90-study. Med Pediatr Oncol. 2001;37:108–14.

Willis B, Ablin A, Weinberg V, Zoger S, Wara WM, Matthay KK. Disease course and late sequelae of Langerhans' cell histiocytosis: 25-year experience at the University of California, San Francisco. J Clin Oncol. 1996;14:2073–82.

Answer to question 108: D

Educational objective

To recognize the causes of marrow fibrosis

Critique

Marrow fibrosis is a reactive process that can be induced by primary hematopoietic stem cell disorders, including any of the myeloproliferative disorders (especially idiopathic myelofibrosis [IMF]), myelodysplastic syndromes (MDS) or acute megakaryoblastic leukemia. Marrow fibrosis can also be induced by infiltrative nonhematopoietic malignancies (e.g. lymphoid and plasma cell neoplasms or metastatic carcinomas), infections (e.g. tuberculosis, atypical mycobacteria or histoplasmosis), metabolic disorders (e.g. Paget disease) or inflammatory/autoimmune disorders (e.g. systemic lupus erythematosus, psoriatic arthritis and primary autoimmune myelofibrosis). Among the potential etiologies, primary autoimmune myelofibrosis is the one disorder that characteristically is not associated with peripheral blood leukoerythroblastic changes and splenomegaly. The other causes of myelofibrosis could produce either or both; however, splenomegaly would be less likely with MDS and metastatic carcinoma, compared with non-Hodgkin lymphoma and IMF. Extreme leukoerythroblastic blood changes and marked splenomegaly would be highly suggestive of IMF, as opposed to the more subtle changes seen with secondary causes of myelofibrosis. Definitive diagnosis in this case requires additional studies to investigate for secondary marrow fibrosis. These would include imaging studies to assess for tumor or lymphadenopathy, marrow immunophenotype analysis to assess for abnormal lymphoid or myeloid populations, and marrow cytogenetics to assess for anomalies consistent with MDS, chronic myeloid leukemia or IMF.

References

Barosi G. Myelofibrosis with myeloid metaplasia. Hematol Oncol Clin North Am. 2003;17:1211–26.

Pullarkat V, Bass RD, Gong JZ, Feinstein DI, Brynes RK. Primary autoimmune myelofibrosis: definition of a distinct clinicopathologic syndrome. Am J Hematol. 2003;72:8–12.

Tefferi A. Myelofibrosis with myeloid metaplasia. N Engl J Med. 2000;342:1255–65.

Answer to question 109: A

Educational objective

To treat myelodysplastic syndrome

Critique

As the only potentially curative therapy, young patients with an appropriate donor should be considered for an allogeneic transplant. Given the relatively young age of this patient, he is more likely to be able to tolerate the potential toxicity of this treatment as well as potentially benefit long term from the procedure. Supportive care is not appropriate for a patient of this age unless all other potentially curative or therapeutic options have been exhausted. In addition, at present there are insufficient data to be able to routinely recommend immunosuppressive therapy outside of a clinical trial. Similarly, there is not enough support in the literature to justify an autologous stem cell transplant for this patient at the present time.

References

Hematology (Am Soc Hematol Educ Program), 2002:136–61.

Luger S, Sacks N. Bone marrow transplantation for myelodysplastic syndrome: who? when? and which? Bone Marrow Transplant. 2002;30:199–206.

Answer to question 110: C

Educational objective

To treat a patient with AML who presents with hyperleukocytosis

Critique

Patients with AML who present with hyperleukocytosis have a life-threatening illness. The primary risk of hyperleukocytosis is leukostasis. Hyperleukocytosis is often associated with early morbidity and mortality. Hyperleukocytosis may be associated with leukocyte thrombi and aggregates within the vasculature. This can occur when the white blood cell count is >100,000/μL. Blood flow in the lungs, brain and other organs may be affected, which may lead to infarction and hemorrhage. In addition, the blasts can compete for oxygen in the microcirculation and invade and damage blood vessels. The immediate objective is to reduce the peripheral blast count rapidly to prevent infarction and hemorrhage. This can be accomplished by leukapheresis, which is an important maneuver, particularly in patients who present with clinical signs and symptoms of leukostasis. In addition, hydroxyurea may also be useful. Leukapheresis is reported to be ineffective and even detrimental in patients with acute promyelocytic leukemia. It is rarely indicated to start chemotherapy until the white blood cell count has been reduced by leukapheresis and hydroxyurea. The role of cranial irradiation is quite controversial. There is potential risk of cerebral hemorrhage.

References

Cuttner J, Holland JF, Norton L. Therapeutic leukapheresis for hyperleukocytosis in acute myelocytic leukemia. Med Pediatr Oncol. 1983;11:76–8.

Grund FM, Armitage JU, Burns CP. Hydroxyurea and the prevention of the effects of leukostasis in acute leukemia. Arch Intern Med. 1977;137:1246–7.

McKee LC, Collins RD. Intravascular leukothrombi and aggregates as a cause of morbidity and mortality in leukemia. Medicine. 1974;53:463–78.

Porcu P, Cripe LD, Ng EW, et al. Hyperleukocytic leukemias and leukostasis: a review of pathophysiology, clinical presentation and management. Leuk Lymphoma. 2000;39:1–18.

Vahdat L, Maslik P, Miller WH Jr, et al. Early mortality and the retinoic acid syndrome in acute promyelocytic leukemia: impact of leukocytosis, low-dose chemotherapy, PML-RAR/α isoform and CD13 expression in patients treated with all-*trans* retinoic acid. Blood. 1994;84:3843–9.

Answer to question 111: E

Educational objective

To identify prognostic factors in adult ALL

Critique

Several factors have been shown to be important prognostic indicators in ALL. Younger age and a low WBC at presentation are favorable, as is the early achievement of complete response (CR) after induction therapy. A fall in circulating blast count to <1000/μL with 1 week of prednisone therapy prior to initiation of induction chemotherapy has been correlated with longer complete response (CR) duration and improved survival. T-cell phenotype had previously been associated with a poorer prognosis, but currently employed multidrug regimens have led to an improved response in T-cell ALL. Cytogenetic analysis often provides prognostic information in both children and adults. The Philadelphia chromosome is present in up to 20% of adult ALL and is associated with a poorer outcome. Other abnormalities associated with an unfavorable outcome include trisomy 8, t(4;11) and t(8;14). Both hyperdiploidy and t(12;21) are associated with a better prognosis. The presence of thrombocytopenia is common and does not have prognostic significance.

References

Thomas X, Le QH. Prognostic factors in adult acute lymphoblastic leukemia. Hematology. 2003;233–42.

Wetzler M. Cytogenetics in adult acute lymphocytic leukemia. Hematol Oncol Clin North Am. 2000;14:1237–49.

Answer to question 112: A

Educational objective

Treatment of early-stage, low-risk Burkitt lymphoma

Critique

Burkitt lymphoma is a highly aggressive non-Hodgkin lymphoma with a high frequency of CNS involvement, even in early-stage disease. Intrathecal chemoprophylaxis is an essential component of induction chemotherapy. Recent intensive combination chemotherapy incorporating high-dose methotrexate has shown improved outcomes, especially in patients such as this with localized low-risk disease (single extra-abdominal mass, normal LDH). Two-year disease-free survival for low-risk patients following three cycles of CODOX-M is reported to be >80%, and so autologous or allogeneic stem cell transplantation in first remission is not routinely recommended.

References

Magrath I, Adde M, Shad A, Venzon D, Seibel N, Gootenberg J, et al. Adults and children with small non-cleaved-cell lymphoma have a similar excellent outcome when treated with the same chemotherapy regimen. J Clin Oncol. 1996;14:1282–90.

Mead GM, Sydes MR, Walewski J, Grigg A, Hatton CS, Norbert P, et al. An international evaluation of CODOX-M and CODOX-M alternating with IVAC in adult Burkitt's lymphoma: results of United Kingdom Lymphoma Group LY06 study. Ann Oncol. 2002;13:1264–74.

Answer to question 113: E

Educational objective

To manage acute venous thromboembolism

Critique

The ventilation perfusion scan is 'high probability' and thus diagnostic of pulmonary embolism. No further testing for acute venous thromboembolism is warranted or required. Inpatient treatment with intravenous unfractionated heparin to achieve a therapeutic activated partial thromboplastin time (APTT), with overlapping warfarin therapy administered to achieve an international normalized ratio (INR) of 2.0–3.0, remains acceptable treatment for acute venous thromboembolism (VTE). Preferred treatment is with outpatient therapeutic dose low-molecular-weight heparin (LMWH), which should be administered in a weight-adjusted dose, according to the manufacturer's recommendations. Recent evidence suggests that long-term LMWH is superior to the combination of initial LMWH followed by warfarin for the prevention of recurrent VTE in patients with active cancer. In any case, the patient should be therapeutically anticoagulated for the rest of his life, as his risk of recurrent VTE would be unacceptably high if anticoagulants were stopped.

References

Lee AY, Levine MN, Baker RI, Bowden C, Kakkar AK, Prins M, et al. Low-molecular-weight heparin versus a coumarin for the prevention of recurrent venous thromboembolism in patients with cancer. N Engl J Med. 2003;349:146–53.

The PIOPED investigators. Value of the ventilation/perfusion scan in acute pulmonary embolism: results of the prospective investigation of pulmonary embolism diagnosis (PIOPED). The PIOPED Investigators. JAMA. 1990;263:2753–9.

Answer to question 114: D

Educational objective

To recognize the risks of viral transmission through transfusion

Critique

Relying upon past teaching or older texts would lead many to answer hepatitis C, but in actuality it is hepatitis B. The risk of transmission of disease by transfusion has changed dramatically since the early 1970s, when post-transfusion hepatitis was linked to the then-common practice of using paid and institutionalized donors with a high carrier rate of hepatitis C. Reliance upon an all-volunteer donor base and the development of HbsAg testing have led to a marked reduction in HCV transmission by transfusion. By the late 1970s and early 1980s, it was recognized that 1 in 10 units was still capable of transmitting post-transfusion non-A, non-B hepatitis (chiefly HCV). Coupled with the growing awareness of the risk of HIV by transfusion, more stringent donor screening and testing measures were initiated throughout the next two decades. After the advent of effective HIV testing in 1985, HCV remained the chief risk until the identification of the virus and the initiation of testing in 1990. Numerous improvements in specific testing for both antigens and antibodies to HIV and the hepatitis viruses have led to extremely low risks. Currently, sensitive PCR-based assays for nucleic acid testing (NAT) are being used to screen for HIV and HCV in transfusion products, with estimates of risk as low as 1 in 1–2 million units. Development of valid NAT for HBV has lagged behind and, even with the use of newer HbsAg tests, the risk of HBV transmission is estimated to be about 1 in 100,000 units. Surface antibody testing cannot be used because of the prevalence of HBV vaccination. There remain donors who are asymptomatic carriers of HBV but have strains that are undetected by both HbsAg and HbcAb testing, and who are not deferred during donor questioning. The relatively low prevalence of HTLV-1/2 infection in US donors and the implementation of antibody screening in the late 1980s have led to an estimated risk of transfusion-acquired HTLV-1/2 as low as 1 in 500,000 units. It was once said by Dr Zuck, the FDA commissioner in the early 1980s, that blood is 'unavoidably unsafe'. Continued concern over emerging risks to the blood supply, such as West Nile virus, SARS virus and certain parasites, are serving as an impetus for the development of sterilization technology for blood products.

References

Dodd RY. Current viral risks of blood and blood products. Ann Med. 2000;32:469–74.

Schreiber GB, Busch MP, Kleinman SH, Korelitz JJ. The risk of transfusion-transmitted viral infections. The Retrovirus Epidemiol Donor Study. N Engl J Med. 1996;334:1685–90.

Weusten JJ, van Drimmelen HA, Lelie PN. Mathematic modeling of the risk of HBV, HCV, and HIV transmission by window-phase donations not detected by NAT. Transfusion. 2002;42:537–48.

Answer to question 115: B

Educational objective

To recognize the features of mantle cell lymphoma

Critique

The immunophenotype is consistent with mantle cell lymphoma. Cyclin D1 is expressed in the majority of patients with mantle cell lymphoma; BCL-6 is typically negative. The translocation associated with mantle cell lymphoma is t(11;14). BCL-6 is expressed in centroblasts, centrocytes, but not by memory B cells, mantle cells and plasma cells. The t(14;18) is associated with follicular lymphoma and the t(2;8) is associated with Burkitt's lymphoma.

References

Decaudin D. Mantle cell lymphoma: a biological and therapeutic paradigm. Leuk Lymphoma. 2002;43:773–81.

Frater J, His ED. Properties of the mantle cell and mantle cell lymphoma. Curr Opin Hematol. 2002;9:56–62.

Answer to question 116: C

Educational objective

To manage heparin-induced thrombocytopenia with thrombosis

Critique

The combination of extending thrombosis coupled with the new onset of thrombocytopenia in a patient recently started on heparin therapy make it imperative to assume the patient has heparin-induced thrombocytopenia with thrombosis (HIT-T) until proven otherwise. An ELISA for heparin-platelet factor 4-dependent antibody may be performed to confirm the diagnosis, but heparin should be stopped and an alternative antithrombotic agent employed without waiting for the result. Two direct thrombin inhibitors, argatroban and lepirudin, are approved for use in this setting. Pentasaccharide has also been shown to be useful, but is not presently FDA-approved. The presence of the cold blue foot makes it likely that the patient also has warfarin-induced venous limb gangrene syndrome, an unintended consequence of the depressive effect of warfarin on protein C synthesis. Heparin must be stopped because the patient has an antibody to platelet-bound heparin that leads to platelet activation and arterial thrombosis. However, the antibody is transient and heparin therapy could be safely used after the antibody disappears generally after 3 months. Warfarin must be stopped until the direct thrombin inhibitor is in the therapeutic range, but may then be safely resumed. Low-molecular-weight heparins can cross-react with heparin-platelet factor 4 antibodies and, thus, are not an appropriate choice for HIT-T.

Reference

Warkentin TE. Heparin-induced thrombocytopenia: pathogenesis and management. Br J Haematol. 2003;121:535–55.

Answer to question 117: C

Educational objective

To recognize procedures to minimize contamination in RT-PCR assays

Critique

Genes are arrayed on chromosomes containing segments that encode protein (exons) separated by segments that do not (introns). Introns vary in length and are often many hundreds of base pairs long. In the process of gene expression, an RNA copy of the gene is made that includes the introns and exons. The introns are spliced out, creating the mature mRNA that is transported to the cytoplasm and translated into protein. RT-PCR is used for the detection and amplification of mRNA from cells. The mRNA is first made into cDNA using reverse transcriptase. The resultant cDNA is then subjected to routine PCR amplification. Often, investigators choose primers for RT-PCR within adjacent exons straddling an intron. Using this design, amplification of cDNA and contaminating genomic products may be differentiated. If the intron is large, the genomic fragment will not be efficiently amplified. The G-C content of the primers chosen will influence the optimal conditions for PCR but will not prevent contamination of the reaction. Because PCR is so sensitive, it is important always to prepare a negative control sample that does not include the template. This type of negative control will not control for the presence of genomic DNA contaminating the cDNA template. Treatment of the RNA with RNAse, before reverse transcription, would destroy the RNA and ruin the experiment. However, the RNA may be treated with RNAse-free DNAse to eliminate contaminating genomic DNA.

Reference

Sambrook J, Russell DW, Sambrook J. Molecular Cloning: A Laboratory Manual. Cold Spring Harbor Laboratory, 15 January, 2001.

Answer to question 118: B

Educational objective

To begin transfusion support in a patient with aplastic anemia

Critique

In patients with aplastic anemia who are stem cell transplant candidates, transfusions should be limited to prevent: (i) sensitization to transplantation antigens; (ii) sensitization to blood antigens; and (iii) cytomegalovirus (CMV) seroconversion. Directed blood products from family members are contraindicated because of reason (i) above. If the patient develops symptomatic cytopenia, transfusion with nonsibling-derived irradiated and leukocyte-depleted blood products is appropriate. Irradiation of the blood products reduces the likelihood of transfusion-related graft-versus-host disease (by compromising the ability of donor leukocytes that contaminate the transfused blood unit to proliferate), and leukocyte depletion decreases the likelihood of allosensitization as well as the risk of transmitting CMV. Erythropoietin and granulocyte colony-stimulating factor injections can be considered but do not constitute standard or effective management of aplastic anemia.

In the context of solid organ transplant, donor-specific blood transfusion pretransplant has been reported to improve organ allograft survival. A proposed mechanism for blood transfusion-mediated improvement in organ survival is the generation of T cells that regulate the immune response (regulatory T cells). The advent of immuno-suppressive drugs such as cyclosporine has diminished any role for donor-specific blood transfusion in the preconditioning of renal allograft recipients. Donor-specific blood transfusion is not a practice that is recommended in bone marrow transplant.

Reference

Otsuka M, Yuzawa K, Takada Y, Taniguchi H, Todoroki K, Fukao K, et al. Long-term results of donor-specific blood transfusion with cyclosporine in living related kidney transplantation. Nephron. 2001;88:144–8.

Answer to question 119: D

Educational objective

To recognize the advantages of pegfilgrastim as an adjunct to myelosuppressive therapy

Critique

The results from several randomized double-blind phase III clinical trials in patients with breast cancer and in patients with lymphoma treated with myelosuppressive chemotherapy have shown that a single dose of pegfilgrastim provides neutrophil support comparable with that provided by an average of 11 days of filgrastim. These studies have also shown that the safety profiles of both cytokines are comparable. Pegfilgrastim given once per cycle may improve patient quality of life because it is easier for patients to receive and results in better compliance with treatment because no doses are missed. The total cost per course is similar between pegfilgrastim and filgrastim.

References

Bohlius J, Reiser M, Schwarzer G, Engert A. Impact of granulocyte colony-stimulating factor (CSF) and granulocyte-macrophage CSF in patients with malignant lymphoma: a systematic review. Br J Haematol. 2003;122:413–23.

Holmes FA, O'Shaughnessy JA, et al. Blinded, randomized, multicenter study to evaluate single administration pegfilgrastim once per cycle versus daily filgrastim as an adjunct to chemotherapy in patients with high risk stage II or stage III/IV breast cancer. J Clin Oncol. 2002;20:727–31.

Vose JM, Crump H, et al. Randomized, multicenter, open-label study of pegfilgrastim compared with daily filgrastim after chemotherapy for lymphoma. J Clin Oncol. 2003;21:514–9.

Answer to question 120: C

Educational objective

To recognize the appropriate treatment for a patient with AIP who presents with uncomplicated abdominal pain

Critique

The most appropriate treatment for a patient with AIP experiencing an acute neurovisceral crisis, such as abdominal pain, consists of caloric loading with dextrose, pain control with narcotic analgesics, and discontinuation of any medications that are known to exacerbate the condition. Surgical consultation is unnecessary as this patient does not have an acute abdomen and has had similar presentations in the past. Panhemitin is indicated with acute respiratory or neurologic decompensation, but not with uncomplicated neurovisceral pain. Psychiatric referral would not be necessary for this patient who has a medical reason for abdominal pain, which is infrequent and does not require excessive narcotic use. Oral contraception has been shown to be associated with clinical flares of neurovisceral symptoms in some patients with AIP and therefore should be discontinued in this patient who had previously been without symptoms for several years.

References

Gonzalez-Arriaza HL, Bostwick JM. Acute porphyrias: a case report and review. Am J Psychiatry. 2003;160:450–9.

Thadani H, Deacon A, Peters T. Diagnosis and management of porphyria. Br Med J. 2000;320:1647–51.

Answer to question 121: (a) A, (b) C

Educational objective

To recognize the cause of megaloblastic anemia and that vitamin B_{12} deficiency may be associated with hyperhomocysteinemia and an increased risk of thrombosis

Critique

As many as 25% of patients with megaloblastic anemia may have an MCV that is within the normal range, although usually it will be within the higher portion of the range and will generally have shown an increase from the patient's healthy state baseline. If left untreated, many patients with megaloblastic anemias will gradually experience pancytopenia. Rarely, patients with megaloblastic states may even present with thrombocytopenia as the first cell line affected in the bone marrow. The hypersegmentation noted on the smear makes cobalamin deficiency the most likely diagnosis of the options presented.

Paroxysmal nocturnal hemoglobinuria (PNH) may be associated with pancytopenia and thrombosis but is not associated with hypersegmentation of neutrophils. While chronic blood loss is a consideration given the low platelets and oral anticoagulation, this would not explain the findings on the peripheral smear. Warm antibody hemolytic anemia and anemia of chronic disease (ACD) would not be associated with the smear findings or with thrombosis. ACD is also unlikely because there is no evidence for a chronic inflammatory condition in this patient, and the very low hemoglobin and high normal MCV would not be typical for ACD.

In the second part to this question, one must recognize the association of high homocysteine blood levels with cobalamin deficiency, and the associated risk of vascular thrombosis. Given the appropriate diagnosis in the first part of the question, hyperhomocysteinemia is the most likely underlying risk factor for thrombosis. Antithrombin deficiency states are rare and generally associated with a strong family history of thrombosis and/or thrombosis presentation at a younger age. PNH is unlikely as determined in the first part of the question. Venous stasis and age over 50 years may augment the risk of hyperhomocysteinemia, but are less significant risk factors for thrombosis than hyperhomocysteinemia.

References

Carmel R. Current concepts in cobalamin deficiency. Annu Rev Med. 2000;51:357–75.

Remecha AF, Souto J, Ramila E, Perea G, Sarda M, Fontcuberta J. Enhanced risk of thrombotic disease in patients with acquired vitamin B_{12} and/or folate deficiency: role of hyperhomocysteinemia. Ann Hematol. 2002;81:616–21.

Answer to question 122: C

Educational objective

To recognize the clinical and laboratory presentation of G6PD deficiency

Critique

This patient presents soon after renal transplant with acute hemolytic anemia and bite cells on the peripheral blood smear. He was started on multiple new medications including trimethoprim-sulfamethoxazole, which is known to increase oxidant stress and may induce episodes of hemolysis in G6PD-deficient individuals. Post-transplant hemolytic uremic syndrome–thrombotic thrombocytopenic purpura (HUS–TTP) is less likely given the normal platelet count, and so stopping cyclosporine or initiating plasma exchange is not warranted. In the African-American variant (A-) of G6PD deficiency, levels should not be sent during the acute crisis as they may be normal secondary to the higher G6PD levels in reticulocytes. Although in the A- variant of G6PD deficiency the drug leading to hemolysis can sometimes be continued if reticulocytosis can be maintained, in this post-transplant patient the drug should be stopped and replaced with another effective agent, such as inhaled pentamidine, which can provide prophylaxis for *Pneumocytis carinii* pneumonia. G6PD deficiency can accurately be diagnosed a few weeks later. Enhancing immunosuppression by increasing the prednisone dose may be indicated in autoimmune hemolytic anemia, but not G6PD deficiency.

References

Beutler E. G6PD deficiency. Blood. 1994;84:3613–36.

Mehta A, Mason PJ, Vulliamy TJ. Glucose-6-phosphate dehydrogenase deficiency. Baillière's Best Pract Res Clin Haematol. 2000;13:21–38.

Answer to question 123: B

Educational objective

To diagnose chronic granulomatous disease

Critique

The patient has clinical features that strongly suggest a defect in neutrophil function. The infectious history, absence of inflammatory signs, slow response to antibiotics and presence of *S. aureus* in a skin abscess support a diagnosis of chronic granulomatous disease (CGD). There is a male preponderance in CGD because the most common molecular lesion is a mutation in the *CYBB* gene, which is located on the X chromosome. Neutrophils from patients with CGD are able to ingest pathogens, but have a defective oxidative burst. The nitroblue tetrazolium (NBT) test is an *in vitro* assay that measures the ability of leukocytes to generate an oxidative burst. The NBT test is much more likely to suggest the correct diagnosis than a bone marrow aspirate, which will show nonspecific reactive changes in the myeloid lineage. Mutations in *SBDS* are found in patients with Schwachman–Diamond syndrome, which is a form of severe congenital neutropenia. This patient does not have neutropenia and the anemia is likely to be secondary to inflammation. The serum ferritin is an unreliable indicator of iron stores in this setting and, in any case, would not be of any use in assessing this patient's propensity to develop infections. A disorder of leukocyte adhesion or migration is a reasonable consideration; however, CGD is much more common and the constellation of clinical findings is most consistent with this possibility. Molecular testing is indicated to characterize the precise mutation in patients with CGD, particularly as gene therapy may emerge as a therapeutic strategy in the next decade. Interferon-γ decreases the incidence and severity of infectious complications in CGD. Patients also require aggressive treatment with antibiotics when they become ill. Hematopoietic stem cell transplantation from an unaffected HLA-matched sibling is a curative treatment for severely affected patients with CGD.

References

Goebel WS, Dinauer MC. Gene therapy for chronic granulomatous disease. Acta Haematol. 2003;110:86–92.

The International Chronic Granulomatous Disease Cooperative Study Group. A controlled trial of interferon-γ to prevent infection in chronic granulomatous disease. N Engl J Med. 1991;324:509–16.

Winkelstein JA, Marino MC, Johnston RB Jr, et al. Chronic granulomatous disease: report on a national registry of 368 patients. Medicine (Baltimore). 2000;79:155–69.

Answer to question 124: B

Educational objective

To treat a patient with advanced idiopathic myelofibrosis

Critique

This patient has developed multiple poor prognostic features for idiopathic myelofibrosis (IMF), including severe anemia, circulating blasts >1%, constitutional symptoms and a new cytogenetic abnormality. With standard supportive management, the median survival at this stage of disease is in the region of 2 years. The left pleural effusion, which is caused by pleural extramedullary hematopoiesis, can be safely and effectively palliated with relatively low-dose radiation (1–1.5 Gy given over 5–10 fractions). Although interferon-α can palliate symptoms and improve cytopenias in some late-stage patients, it could also cause significant side-effects or worsen cytopenias. Thalidomide, with or without prednisone, would be a more tolerable treatment option for the cytopenias and massive splenomegaly; however, this agent would likely not control the pleural effusion. A myeloablative hematopoietic stem cell transplant from the HLA-matched sister provides the only definitive and potentially curative treatment for this patient with late-stage disease. The 2-year survival rates after myeloablative transplant, from single-institution experience, are approximately 40–58%, with the highest survival and lowest mortality among those patients transplanted earlier in their disease course. Morbidity and mortality may be minimized, particularly in older patients, by using targeted-dose conditioning chemotherapy and donor peripheral blood stem cells (rather than marrow).

References

Daly A, Song K, Nevill T, Nantel S, Toze C, Hogge D, et al. Stem cell transplantation for myelofibrosis: a report from two Canadian centers. Bone Marrow Transplant. 2003;32:35–40.

Deeg HJ, Gooley TA, Flowers MED, Sale GE, Slattery JT, Anasetti C, et al. Allogeneic hematopoietic stem cell transplantation for myelofibrosis. Blood. 2003;102:3912–8.

Koch CA, Li CY, Mesa RA, Tefferi A. Nonhepatosplenic extramedullary hematopoiesis: associated diseases, pathology, clinical course, and treatment. Mayo Clin Proc. 2003;78:1223–33.

Answer to question 125: C

Educational objective

To treat chronic myelomonocytic leukemia

Critique

The World Health Organization (WHO) has classified chronic myelomonocytic leukemia (CMML) along with atypical CML and juvenile myelomonocytic leukemia in a myelodysplastic/myeloproliferative overlap category. Therapeutic choices typically depend on the predominant form of the disease and the disease features that predominate. Some CMML patients with proliferative features may require hydroxyurea to control proliferation and allow for improved hematopoiesis, while others may require transfusion support for symptomatic cytopenias. A small percentage of patients with CMML and the t(5;12) may respond to imatinib mesylate. This tyrosine kinase inhibitor can specifically inhibit platelet-derived growth factor receptor β (PDGFRB) which is activated in patients with the t(5;12). Imatinib can induce a clinical and cytogenetic remission in patients with CMML and this cytogenetic abnormality.

Reference

Apperley JF, Gardembas M, Melo JV, Russell-Jones R, Bain BJ, Baxter EJ, et al. Response to imatinib mesylate in patients with chronic myeloproliferative diseases with rearrangements of platelet-derived growth factor receptor β. N Engl J Med. 2002;347:481–7.

Answer to question 126: E

Educational objective

To recognize and treat the retinoic acid syndrome

Critique

Acute promyelocytic leukemia is treated differently from all other subtypes of AML and has emerged as the most curable subtype. A major advance has been the introduction of the vitamin A derivative, all-*trans* retinoic acid (ATRA). The most important complication of ATRA is a cardiorespiratory distress syndrome called the retinoic acid syndrome. This is manifested by interstitial pulmonary infiltrates, pleural or pericardial effusions, hypoxemia and episodic hypertension, with otherwise unexplained weight gain. The syndrome may be, but is not always, associated with the rapid development of hyperleukocytosis. The sydrome resolves quickly if corticosteroids are administered at the very earliest sign of symptoms. The standard practice is to administer dexamethasone 10 mg twice daily for 3 days. If the syndrome is severe, it is routine practice to temporarily discontinue ATRA until the syndrome has resolved. There is no indication to introduce additional chemotherapy.

References

De Botton BS, Dombret H, Sanz M, et al. Incidence, clinical features, and outcome of all-*trans* retinoic acid syndrome in 413 cases of newly diagnosed acute promyelocytic leukemia. The European APL Group. Blood. 1998;92:2712–8.

Tallman MS, Andersen JW, Schiffer CA, et al. Clinical description of 44 patients with acute promyelocytic leukemia who developed the retinoic acid syndrome. Blood. 2000;95:90–5.

Answer to question 127: B

Educational objective

To recognize treatment components of adult ALL

Critique

Improvements in the outcome of adult ALL have occurred with protocols similar to those used in pediatric ALL. Multiple cycles of intensive multiagent chemotherapy are important, as are intrathecal prophylaxis and maintenance (continuation) therapy. With initial induction therapy, patients are at high risk of tumor lysis and require aggressive treatment and monitoring. Consolidation therapy with high-dose cytarabine as the only post-induction therapy would be appropriate for acute myeloid leukemia, but would not be adequate for ALL.

Reference

Hoelzer D, Gokbuget N, Ottmann O, Pui C.-H, Relling MV, Appelbaum FR, et al. Acute lymphoblastic leukemia. Hematology. 2002;162–92.

Answer to question 128: D

Educational objective

To treat advanced-stage Hodgkin disease

Critique

The current standard chemotherapy for advanced-stage Hodgkin lymphoma (stage IIB-IV) is ABVD chemotherapy. Randomized studies over the last 15 years have demonstrated similar activity between ABVD and MOPP or MOPP/ABV hybrid regimens, but with less acute and chronic toxicity. The standard is at least six cycles, or two cycles past best response up to eight cycles. Subsequent radiation therapy is recommended to sites of disease >10 cm because of increased risk of local relapse. Reduced cycles of multiagent chemotherapy with involved field radiation are active for early-stage disease (stage I and II), but are not recommended for advanced-stage and bulky disease. Although high-dose therapy appears to have a role in the treatment of patients with relapsed disease, it has not been shown to benefit patients as part of initial therapy. Similarly, the routine use of radiation is not indicated in patients with advanced-stage, nonbulky disease, although it may have a role for those patients with a partial response to chemotherapy. Comparative trials of ABVD versus the BEACOPP or Stanford V regimens are in progress for patients with advanced-stage disease and unfavorable risk factors.

References

Connors JM, Noordijk EM, Horning SJ. Hodgkin's Lymphoma: Basing the treatment on the evidence. Hematology. 2001;178–93.

Diehl V, Stein H, Hummel M, Zollinger R, Connors JM. Hodgkin's lymphoma: biology and treatment strategies for primary, refractory and relapsed disease. Hematology. 2003; 225–47.

Answer to question 129: C

Educational objective

To diagnose the causes of treatment failure in stem cell transplant for nonmalignant diseases

Critique

Children with nonmalignant disorders frequently can be cured by stem cell transplant. The difficulty is that many of these children have affected siblings with less dramatic presentations of the same disorder. It is important to evaluate the donor for the possibility of the same disease. The possibility of HUS–TTP exists; however, this patient's platelets were normal. The possibility of graft failure that is selective to red cells only is unlikely. The timing of the fall in counts does not correspond with the development of MDS and the donor is a child who is not likely to have the condition. The possibility of hemolysis secondary to different blood types exists but this generally results in mild anemia without the need for ongoing transfusions.

Reference

Gaziev J, Lucarelli G. Stem cell transplantation for hemoglobinopathies. Curr Opin Pediatr. 2003;15:24–31.

Answer to question 130: D

Educational objective

To recognize factor XII deficiency

Critique

A normal INR and prolonged APTT are diagnostic of a factor deficiency in the intrinsic coagulation cascade. Deficiencies of factors VIII or IX sufficient to cause an APTT >150 s would be associated with a profound hemorrhagic diathesis, particularly with scoliosis surgery. Factor XI deficiency may not cause bleeding; however, it is unlikely that a factor XI deficiency would either cause an APTT prolongation of this magnitude or not be associated with bleeding with scoliosis surgery. Factor XIII deficiency does not cause a prolonged APTT. Severe deficiency of factor XII is relatively common compared with other coagulation factor deficiencies, is frequently associated with an APTT >150 s, and is not associated with a bleeding diathesis. The diagnosis is confirmed with appropriate coagulation factor levels.

Reference

Lammle WA, Wuillemin I, Huber M, Krauskopf C, Zurcher R, Pflugshaupt M, et al. Thromboembolism and bleeding tendency in congenital factor XII deficiency: a study on 74 subjects from 14 Swiss families. Thromb Haemost. 1991;65:117–21.

Answer to question 131: D

Educational objective

To recognize the clinical features and diagnostic problems of drug-induced thrombocytopenia

Critique

A drug-induced etiology of thrombocytopenia may often be unrecognized, especially in patients who have been previously diagnosed with ITP or another disorder associated with thrombocytopenia. In this patient, the previous diagnosis of ITP suggested that his recurrent episodes of thrombocytopenia were caused by recurrent ITP. However, ITP in adults is typically a persistent disorder, often poorly or slowly responsive to treatment; ITP does not characteristically cause repeated sudden severe thrombocytopenia followed by prompt recovery. This patient very likely continued to take quinine tablets intermittently, because patients often continue medicines that they regulate themselves and take only occasionally, and often assume that their doctor does not deem these medicines to be important. The clue here is the history of musculoskeletal symptoms, and therefore the most likely etiology for the thrombocytopenia is quinine taken for muscle cramps. Quinine is currently the most common cause of drug-induced thrombocytopenia and patients will usually assume that doctors are not interested in quinine when they ask about medications. Thus, questions asking specifically about quinine, and tonic water, are essential.

The course of thrombocytopenia is not suggestive of recurrent ITP, and therefore treatment with rituximab or evaluation for an accessory spleen is not appropriate. Thrombocytopenia associated with non-Hodgkin lymphoma is comparable to ITP and also unlikely. Recurrent episodes of TTP are an intriguing consideration, as TTP may be misdiagnosed as ITP and some patients may recover without plasma exchange treatment. However, to have three episodes within 4 weeks without recognition of systemic symptoms or overt hemolysis is unlikely.

References

George JN, Raskob GE, Shah SR, Rizvi MA, Hamilton SA, Osborne S, et al. Drug-induced thrombocytopenia: a systematic review of published case reports. Ann Intern Med. 1998;129:886–90.

Kojouri K, Perdue JJ, George JN. Occult quinine-induced thrombocytopenia. J Okla State Med Assoc. 2000;93:519–21.

Neylon AJ, Saunders PWG, Howard MR, Proctor SJ, Taylor PRA. Clinically significant newly presenting autoimmune thrombocytopenic purpura in adults: a prospective study of a population-based cohort of 245 patients. Br J Haematol. 2003;122:966–74.

Answer to question 132: D

Educational objective

To treat childhood neuroblastoma

Critique

Based on the location of the tumor, the child's age and the histologic description of the tumor, the patient is most likely to have a neuroblastoma. She has stage IV disease. This tumor appears to be responsive to high-dose chemotherapy. A randomized trial by the Children's Cancer Group (CCG) demonstrated an advantage to reduction of the disease burden to no evidence of reduction (NED) followed by high-dose chemotherapy with autologous rescue. Timing of treatment aimed at local reduction of the primary tumor may vary from center to center but generally requires surgery and/or radiation. Various centers process the stem cells differently—some purge using an antibody directed against a neuroblastoma epitope while others $CD34^+$ select. Differentiation therapy with 13-*cis*-retinoic acid for 6 months follows the transplant. Allogeneic transplant has not been proven to have a benefit in the treatment of neuroblastoma.

Reference

Matthay KK, Villablanca JG, Seeger RC, Stram DO, Harris RE, Ramsay NK, et al. Treatment of high-risk neuroblastoma with intensive chemotherapy, radiotherapy, autologous bone marrow transplantation, and 13-*cis*-retinoic acid. Children's Cancer Group. N Engl J Med. 1999;341:1165–73.

Answer to question 133: B

Educational objective

To recognize the hemolytic anemia in passenger lymphocyte syndrome

Critique

The most likely diagnosis is hemolysis brought about by the passenger lymphocyte syndrome. The likelihood of the diagnosis is increased because the syndrome occurred 2–3 weeks after transplant, the donor is type O and the recipient is type A, and direct antibody test is positive for an IgG antibody. Immunocompetent donor B lymphocytes have been shown to be transplanted as 'passengers' in the donor liver and are subsequently capable of producing hemolytic antibodies against red cell antigens not present in the donor; in this case, the common A antigen. Subjects who are ABO/Rh compatible can develop passenger lymphocyte-associated hemolytic anemia related to incompatibility of minor blood group antigens. The episode of hemolysis is usually limited to a few weeks. Because the donor was Rh-positive, anti-Rh antibodies would not be expected. Panagglutinins, typical of autoimmune hemolytic anemia, and cold agglutinins, usually IgM and not hemolytic, have not been described in the passenger lymphocyte syndrome.

Reference

Sokol RJ, Stamps R, Booker DJ, Scott FM, Laidlaw ST, Vandenberghe EA, et al. Post transplant immune-mediated hemolysis. Transfusion. 2002;42:198–204.

Answer to question 134: D

Educational objective

To recognize the mechanism of transfusion-related acute lung injury

Critique

This patient experienced respiratory distress and hypoxemia 2 h after transfusion, with low-grade fever and evidence of pulmonary edema. Transfusion-related acute lung injury (TRALI) is a pathophysiologic mechanism attributed to the effect of leukoagglutinins (alloantibodies reactive against leukocyte antigens) of donor origin that cause activation of granulocytes in the pulmonary capillary bed when the recipient's leukocytes express the antigen recognized by the antibody. TRALI is chiefly seen after transfusion of plasma products such as platelets or fresh frozen plasma (FFP) that contain sufficient amounts of the donor antibody, although high-titer leukoagglutinins have been implicated in TRALI cases arising from red cell units. It takes some time for the leukocyte activation to become symptomatic, and TRALI often presents hours after the transfusion. If the reaction is severe, acute respiratory distress syndrome (ARDS) may develop. It is sometimes difficult to distinguish the symptomatology of TRALI from antibody-mediated febrile nonhemolytic transfusion reactions (FNHTR), which are also caused by leukoagglutinins, although in FNHTR the antibody is of recipient origin directed against transfused donor leukocytes. Just as there are cytokine-mediated cases of FNHTR that are not caused by leukoagglutinins, some cases of TRALI have been attributed to putative leukocyte-activating substances in stored blood products when leukoagglutinins could not be detected. While reactions from bacterial contamination of platelets can cause respiratory distress, these are usually manifested by high fever and hypotension, and pulmonary edema is a late finding. Anaphylaxis would present with signs of hypotension and mucosal edema, and often patients have other allergic symptoms such as rash or hives. While acute hemolytic reactions can lead to respiratory distress, these are usually more immediate. The group AB platelets in this case would not contain anti-B and apheresis platelets have little red cell contamination, making ABO incompatibility, capable of causing these symptoms, unlikely. Circulatory overload from transfusion can cause respiratory distress, but is most often seen in the very young or the very old, or in patients with significant cardiovascular compromise. In addition, circulatory overload causes plethora and blood pressure elevation, and does not cause fever.

References

Kopko PM, Paglieroni TG, Popovsky MA, Muto KN, MacKenzie MR, Holland PV. TRALI: correlation of antigen–antibody and monocyte activation in donor–recipient pairs. Transfusion. 2003;43:177–84.

Silliman CC, Boshkov LK, Mehdizadehkashi Z, Elzi DJ, Dickey WO, Podlosky L, et al. Transfusion-related acute lung injury: epidemiology and a prospective analysis of etiologic factors. Blood. 2003;101:454–62.

Wallis JP. Transfusion-related acute lung injury (TRALI): under-diagnosed and under-reported. Br J Anaesth. 2003;90:573–6.

Answer to question 135: A

Educational objective

To recognize the cytogenetic abnormalities in leukemia associated with topoisomerase II inhibitor therapy

Critique

Topoisomerase II inhibitor-related leukemias are most frequently monocytic or myelomonocytic. This type of leukemia is usually not preceded by a myelodysplastic phase. The median time between drug exposure and acute leukemia is 34 months. The two classes of drugs most often implicated are the epipodophyllotoxins and the anthracyclines. The predominant cytogenetic finding is a balanced translocation or a deletion involving 11q23. The *MLL* gene on 11q23 is involved in the translocations or deletions. Butyrate esterase is positive in monocytes and monoblasts. The inv(16) (p13;q22) is most frequently associated with acute myelomonocytic leukemia with eosinophilia. The inv(3) (q21;q26) is seen in acute megakaryocytic leukemia. The t(11;17)(q13;q21) is an acute promyelocytic leukemia variant translocation.

References

Jaffe ES, Harris NL, Stein H, Vardiman JW. WHO Tumours of Haematopoietic and Lymphoid Tissues. Lyon: IARC Press, 2001.

Smith SM, Le beau MM, Huo D, Karrison T, Sobecks RM, Anastasi J, et al. Clinical–cytogenetic associations in 306 patients with therapy-related myelodysplasia and myeloid leukemia: the University of Chicago series. Blood. 2003;102:43–52.

Answer to question 136: D

Educational objective

To recognize and appropriately manage ITP in pregnancy

Critique

The most likely diagnosis is chronic idiopathic thrombocytopenic purpura (ITP) based on the clinical pattern of chronic fluctuating thrombocytopenia in the absence of symptoms and signs in a young woman. Studies of pregnant women with ITP have reported no evidence that the level of maternal platelet count is related to the platelet count of the fetus or newborn. The risk to this patient's fetus is relatively low because the mother has an intact spleen and a platelet count of 50,000/μL, and has previously delivered two normal infants following pregnancies with thrombocytopenia. Medicating the mother with prednisone or IVIG would not benefit the fetus and is not indicated for the mother. Funipuncture should only be considered in a center in which it is a standard procedure and then only if the platelet count fell below 50,000/μL and the mother was symptomatic. The decision to perform funipuncture should be made if, and only if, the level of fetal thrombocytopenia would guide clinical management at delivery, and should not be considered a routine management plan early in pregnancy. Cesarean section has not been shown to provide a benefit to the fetus. Infants born to mothers with ITP usually have normal platelet counts, although the fetal platelet count may drop precipitously on the third or fourth day of life. Cerebral hemorrhage is a rare complication of vaginal delivery even for neonates born with ITP. Causes of thrombocytopenia other than ITP might be considered, for example TTP–HUS, DIC, HELLP syndrome with pre-eclampsia and folate deficiency. None of these seem likely in the context of asymptomatic thrombocytopenia with prolonged chronicity.

Reference

Webert KE, Mittal R, Sigouin C, Heddle NM, Kelton JG. A retrospective 11-year analysis of obstetric patients with idiopathic thrombocytopenic purpura. Blood. 2003;102:4306.

Answer to question 137: C

Educational objective

To recognize procedures for prenatal diagnosis of factor VIII deficiency

Critique

Hemophilia A is a genetically heterogeneous disorder. It is rarely caused by a point mutation. Approximately 40% of individuals with severe hemophilia A carry a large inversion of the factor VIII gene. This inversion may be detected by Southern blot analysis. Prenatal diagnosis is facilitated by knowledge of the factor VIII abnormality that is present in the family. Hemophilia A is an X-linked disorder. Prenatal diagnostic studies are usually restricted to male fetuses. Genetic studies may be performed earlier in gestation, with more diagnostic precision and with less risk than umbilical blood sampling.

References

Cao A, Galanello R, Rosatelli MC. Prenatal diagnosis and screening of the haemoglobinopathies. Baillière's Clin Haematol. 1998;11:215–38.

Lakich D, Kazazian HH Jr, Antonarakis SE, et al. Inversions disrupting the factor VIII gene are a common cause of severe haemophilia A. Nat Genet. 1993;5:236–41.

Answer to question 138: B

Educational objective

To treat severe aplastic anemia in a patient <40 years of age

Critique

This patient's age (<40 years) and disease severity fall within the range in which stem cell transplant from a fully matched sibling donor is the first choice treatment for severe aplastic anemia.

After conditioning with cyclophosphamide, 90% of stem cell grafts from HLA-identical siblings successfully engraft in patients who have not received transfusions; 80–90% of these patients achieve long-term survival with normal hematopoietic function. In patients with transfusion-induced sensitization to transplantation antigens, cyclophosphamide alone results in a high incidence of graft rejection (30%) and decreased survival rates (40–50%) unless more intensive conditioning is administered. Sensitization to transplantation antigens can occur after any number of transfusions but is more likely after approximately 30 units of red cells. To improve the success with engraftment in sensitized patients, high-dose cyclophosphamide and ATG conditioning has resulted in a 92% survival rate as compared with the 72% survival rate of a historical cohort of patients conditioned with cyclophosphamide alone. Cyclophosphamide together with limited field irradiation also improves engraftment but there is a higher incidence of secondary malignancies, infertility and, in children, retardation of growth and development.

Reference

Deeg HJ, Leisenring W, Storb R, et al. Long-term outcome after marrow transplantation for severe aplastic anemia. Blood. 1998;91:3637–45.

Answer to question 139: C

Educational objective

To differentiate variegate porphyria from other porphyric syndromes

Critique

This patient of Dutch heritage has a personal and family history of neurovisceral symptoms and blistering skin lesions, consistent with the diagnosis of variegate porphyria. Fecal protoporphyrins could be collected to confirm the diagnosis. Skin lesions are not present in AIP and neurovisceral symptoms are not present in porphyria cutanea tarda. Congenital erythropoietic porphyria is extremely rare and leads to ulcerative skin lesions, anemia and skeletal changes.

References

Gonzalez-Arriaza HL, Bostwick JM. Acute porphyrias: a case report and review. Am J Psychiatry. 2003;160:450–9.

Thadani H, Deacon A, Peters T. Diagnosis and management of porphyria. Br Med J. 2000;320:1647–51.

Answer to question 140: D

Educational objective

To recognize laboratory features consistent with common causes of anemia in HIV-infected patients

Critique

HIV patients maintained on AZT therapy will have an elevated MCV that can occur with or without anemia. Elevated MCV determinations are followed as a way of assessing patients' compliance in taking their medication. In HIV-infected individuals, chronic bone marrow suppression leading to anemia with inappropriate reticulocyte response can occur with chronic parvovirus, AZT (and other antiretrovirals) and direct bone marrow infection with fungal and mycobacterial organisms.

While TTP does occur with increased frequency in association with HIV infection, expected findings would include abnormal renal function tests as well as signs of intravascular hemolysis such as a high LDH and low haptoglobin. Many patients with HIV-associated TTP will not be able to mount a good reticulocyte response because of other causes of marrow suppression as noted above.

References

Bain B. Pathogenesis and pathophysiology of anemia in HIV infection. Curr Opin Hematol. 1999;6:89–93.

Koduri PR. Parvovirus B19-related anemia in HIV-infected patients. AIDS Patient Care Stds. 2000;14:7–11.

Sullivan P, Hanson D, Chu S, Jones J, Ward J. Epidemiology of anemia in human immunodeficiency virus (HIV) infected persons: results from the multistate adult and adolescent spectrum of HIV disease surveillance project. Blood. 1998;91:301–8.

Answer to question 141: B

Educational objective

To recognize and evaluate an aplastic crisis in a patient with a chronic hemolytic anemia

Critique

This patient likely has hereditary spherocytosis based on his peripheral blood smear, previously elevated reticulocyte count, history of gallstones and family history. He now presents with an acute severe hypoproliferative anemia after exposure to a child with a rash. The etiology of the childhood illness and the aplastic crisis is likely parvovirus B19, which can be diagnosed by PCR testing of DNA. An osmotic fragility test would not provide the diagnosis for the acute drop in hematocrit and reticulocytopenia, but could be performed later to assess for hereditary spherocytosis. A direct antiglobulin test (DAT) would be useful if autoimmune hemolytic anemia was the likely diagnosis. A primary marrow disorder would be unlikely given the acuity of the anemia and the maintenance of a normal white blood cell and platelet count.

References

Bolton-Maggs PH. The diagnosis and management of hereditary spherocytosis. Best Pract Res Clin Haematol. 2000;13:327–42.

Skinnider LF, McSheffrey BJ, Sheridan D, Deneer H. Congenital spherocytic hemolytic anemia in a family presenting with transient red cell aplasia from parvovirus B19 infection. Am J Hematol. 1998;58:341–2.

Smith JC, Megason GC, Iyer RV, Andrew ME, Pullen DJ. Clinical characteristics of children with hereditary hemolytic anemias and aplastic crisis: a 7-year review. South Med J. 1994;87:702–8.

Answer to question 142: C

Educational objective

To treat a patient with chronic myeloid leukemia (CML) in early chronic phase

Critique

This patient has come to you to decide which treatment course to pursue. He has a matched sibling donor and would clearly belong to the group that has the best long-term disease-free survival with a myeloablative allogeneic stem cell transplant. Successful myeloablative transplantation will eradicate the malignant clone and offer this patient a chance for cure, not to prolong his chronic phase. His chance of long-term survival is >60% and in some studies as high as 85% if he undergoes a matched related donor allogeneic transplantation. There are no long-term data for imatinib and so it cannot be directly compared with allogeneic transplantation. Transplantation following nonmyeloablative conditioning has shown efficacy but has not been directly compared with myeloablative approaches. However, many patients are choosing to be treated with imatinib and it remains to be seen if patients will do as well long term.

References

Melo JV, Hughes TP, Apperley JF. Chronic myeloid leukemia. Hematology (Am Soc Hematol Educ Program) 2003:132–52.

Wayne AS, Barrett AJ. Allogeneic hematopoietic stem cell transplantation for myeloproliferative disorders and myelodysplastic syndromes. Hematol Oncol Clin North Am. 2003;17:1175–90.

Weisdorf DJ, Anasetti C, Antin JH, Kernan NA, Kollman C, Snyder D, et al. Allogeneic bone marrow transplantation for chronic myelogenous leukemia: comparative analysis of unrelated versus matched sibling donor transplantation. Blood. 2002;99:1971–7.

Answer to question 143: E

Educational objective

To recognize clinical and biologic features of juvenile myelomonocytic leukemia

Critique

This patient has a 'classic' constellation of findings that support a diagnosis of juvenile myelomonocytic leukemia (JMML). Boys are affected much more often than girls—this male predilection is present in children who develop JMML in the context of a genetic predisposition such as neurofibromatosis type 1 (as in this case) or Noonan syndrome. Children with Fanconi anemia are at increased risk of developing MDS and AML, but not JMML. Cell culture and cytogenetic studies can provide important additional diagnostic information. A hallmark of JMML is a selective pattern of hypersensitive growth in response to the growth factor GM-CSF. Monosomy 7 is a frequent cytogenetic finding that would also support this diagnosis. Whereas bone marrow hypercellularity, morphologic dysplasia and peripheral cytopenias are classic features of MDS, children with JMML present with a mixed pattern of dysplasia in association with prominent myeloproliferation. Adults with CMML and atypical CML show similar findings. As a result, the new category of myelodysplastic/myeloproliferative disorder was developed by the WHO group, which includes CMML, JMML and atypical CML. The prognosis is poor in JMML, with very few patients cured without transplantation.

References

Arico M, Biondi A, Pui C-H. Juvenile myelomonocytic leukemia. Blood. 1997;90:479–88.

Emanuel PD, Shannon KM, Castleberry RP. Juvenile myelomonocytic leukemia: molecular understanding and prospects for therapy. Mol Med Today. 1996;2:468–75.

Answer to question 144: B

Educational objective

To recognize optimal therapy for secondary AML

Critique

Patients with secondary AML have an unfavorable prognosis. Two general subtypes have been described. The first type of secondary AML is associated with alkylating agent exposure. This subtype usually has a relatively long latency period and often an antecedent period of myelodysplasia. Leukemia cells may demonstrate abnormalities in chromosomes 5 and 7, monosomy 5 or 7, or 5q- or 7q-. The second type of secondary AML is associated with prior exposure to topoisomerase II targeting agents, such as the epipodophyllotoxins and the anthracyclines. The characteristic karyotype abnormality is the presence of a translocation involving chromosome band 11q23. Molecular studies often show rearrangement of the *MLL* (mixed lineage leukemia) gene. There is no evidence that administering a more intensive induction program to patients with secondary AML is of benefit.

Patients with poor-risk cytogenetics may fare better with a transplant procedure that induces a graft-versus-leukemia effect, as opposed to consolidation chemotherapy alone. A fully ablative allogeneic stem cell transplant is more likely than a nonmyeloablative transplant to produce clinically significant graft-versus-host disease. There is a fair correlation of graft-versus-host disease with an antileukemia effect in patients with AML. However, graft-versus-host disease carries an increased risk of morbidity and mortality, especially in older individuals. There is no evidence for a benefit of autologous stem cell transplantation. If a younger patient (age <60 years) with secondary AML has a suitably matched sibling donor, many would recommend proceeding with a myeloablative stem cell transplant following induction (with or without a course of consolidation chemotherapy). It may also be reasonable to consider a matched unrelated donor stem cell transplant in even younger patients (age <40 years).

References

van Leeuwen FE. Risk of acute myelogenous leukemia myelodysplasia following cancer treatment. Ballière's Clin Haematol. 1996;9:57–85.

Pedersen-Bjergaard J. Radiotherapy- and chemotherapy-induced myelodysplasia in acute myeloid leukemia: a review. Leuk Res. 1992;16:61–5.

Pui C-H, Roberio RC, Hancock ML, et al. Acute myeloid leukemia in children treated with epipodophyllotoxins for acute lymphoblastic leukemia. N Engl J Med. 1991;325:1682–7.

Sierra J, Store RB, Hansen JA, et al. Unrelated donor marrow transplantation for acute myeloid leukemia: an update of the Seattle experience. Bone Marrow Transplant. 2000;26:397–404.

Slovak ML, Kopecky KJ, Cassileth PA, et al. Karyotypic analysis predicts outcome of preremission and postremission therapy in adult acute myeloid leukemia: a Southwest Oncology Group/Eastern Cooperative Oncology Group Study. Blood. 2000;96:4075–83.

Answer to question 145: B

Educational objective

To recognize the prognostic significance of cytogenetic findings in multiple myeloma

Critique

The degree of plasmacytosis on bone marrow biopsy, anemia, lytic bone lesions and renal insufficiency are important criteria for differentiating multiple myeloma from monoclonal gammopathy of undetermined significance (MGUS) or smoldering myeloma and for classifying by stage. However, they do not have significant prognostic impact. Other factors that can help predict outcome include the measurement of the number of plasma cells in S phase, and cytogenetics. The S-phase fraction correlates with the rate of division of plasma cells and has been shown to strongly predict outcome, but is not widely available. Although conventional cytogenetics is often difficult in plasma cell disorders because of its reliance on dividing cells, the use of FISH and other techniques has detected recurring defects in multiple myeloma. These include deletions of chromosomes 13 and 17 and translocations involving chromosomes 11 and 14. In a study by Shaughnessy et al., deletions of chromosome 13 were associated with a poorer outcome.

References

Barlogie B, Shaughnessy J, Tricot G, et al. Treatment of multiple myeloma. Blood. 2004;103:20–32.

Durie B, Stock-Novack D, Salmon SE, Finley P, Beckord J, Crowley J, Coltman CA. Prognostic value of pretreatment serum β_2-microglobulin in myeloma: a Southwest Oncology Group Study. Blood. 1990;75:823–30.

Shaughnessy J, Tian E, Sawyer J, et al. Prognostic impact of cytogenetic and interphase fluorescence *in situ* hybridization-defined chromosome 13 deletion in multiple myeloma: early results of total therapy II. Br J Haematol. 2003;120:44–52.

Answer to question 146: E

Educational objective

To identify the appropriate source of stem cells for children

Critique

In the USA, children with AML who obtain remission following induction chemotherapy and have a matched family donor are transplanted in first complete remission. This is largely because of the low rate of preparative regimen toxicity in good risk patients such as these. Early transplantation is chosen over the watchful waiting approach used in most standard risk AML adult patients. Stem cells from an available donor will be selected over a cord blood product at most institutions because of the ability to obtain an adequate stem cell dose, but also because of the lack of graft-versus-leukemia effect in cord blood products. The patient's sister is haplo-identical and would not be considered as a donor given the availability of another HLA-identical sibling. The cord blood from his sister could be used if no alternative donor was available. Autologous transplant in this case has no role because of the factors discussed above: the generation of a graft-versus-leukemia effect from an allogeneic donor and the low morbidity and mortality associated with matched sibling transplants in young children. Attempts to purge autologous bone marrow products have frequently resulted in prolonged neutropenia.

References

Neudorf S, Sanders J, Kobrinsky N, Alonzo TA, Buxton AB, Gold S, et al. Allogeneic bone marrow transplantation for children with acute myelocytic leukemia in first remission demonstrates a role for graft versus leukemia in the maintenance of disease-free survival. Blood. 2004;103:3655–61.

Woods WG, Neudorf S, Gold S, Sanders J, Buckley JD, Barnard DR, et al. Children's Cancer Group. A comparison of allogeneic bone marrow transplantation, autologous bone marrow transplantation, and aggressive chemotherapy in children with acute myeloid leukemia in remission. Blood. 2001;97:56–62.

Answer to question 147: D

Educational objective

To recognize therapy that reduces mortality in patients with severe sepsis

Critique

There is no evidence that heparin therapy ameliorates either the development or clinical course of disseminated intravascular coagulopathy (DIC). Its use should, in general, be confined to patients with objectively confirmed micro- or macrovascular thrombosis. Large studies have examined the efficacy of TFPI, AT or rAPC in patients with severe sepsis. In these studies, only rAPC therapy was associated with a reduction in mortality. Thrombolytic therapy may exacerbate sepsis-associated coagulopathy and should be avoided.

References

Abraham E, Reinhart K, Opal S, Demeyer I, Doig C, Rodriguez AL, et al. Efficacy and safety of tifacogin (recombinant tissue factor pathway inhibitor) in severe sepsis: a randomized controlled trial. JAMA. 2003;290:238–47.

Bernard GR, Vincent JL, Laterre PF, LaRosa SP, Dhainaut JF, Lopez-Rodriguez A, et al. Efficacy and safety of recombinant human activated protein C for severe sepsis. N Engl J Med. 2001;344:699–709.

Warren BL, Eid A, Singer P, Pillay SS, Carl P, Novak I, et al. Caring for the critically ill patient: high-dose antithrombin III in severe sepsis—a randomized controlled trial. JAMA. 2001;286:1869–78.

Answer to question 148: E

Educational objective

To recognize a cytokine-mediated febrile reaction

Critique

This patient experienced fever and rigors during a transfusion, and is having a typical febrile nonhemolytic transfusion reaction (FNHTR). Classically, these were attributed to leukoagglutinins of recipient origin directed against transfused donor white cells, and were seen predominantly in patients alloimmunized through pregnancy or previous transfusion. Leukocyte reduction by methods as inefficient as buffy coat removal, which achieves at best a two-log reduction in the leukocyte content of a unit of red cells, can reduce the incidence of these reactions. However, this male patient does not have a history of previous transfusion, and so is not at risk of having leukoagglutinins. This underscores perhaps the more common mechanism that causes FNHTR. Cytokines derived from donor leukocytes that become activated during blood storage can also produce the symptoms of an FNHTR. Even modern bedside leukocyte filters, which can reduce the leukocyte content below 10^6 WBC, will not prevent these reactions if the leukocytes activate and release these cytokines during storage. This has been one of the stimuli to achieve universal prestorage leukoreduction. The lack of hypotension and the transfusion of red cells rather than platelets make bacterial contamination an unlikely cause. Although the symptoms were seen relatively soon after starting the transfusion, they cannot be confused with anaphylaxis, which does not cause fever. The lack of signs or symptoms of hemolysis and negative direct antiglobulin test make an acute transfusion reaction unlikely. His gender and lack of previous transfusion exposure make it unlikely he has alloantibodies against donor leukocytes.

References

Heddle NM. Pathophysiology of febrile nonhemolytic transfusion reactions. Curr Opin Hematol. 1999;6:420–6.

Perrotta PL, Snyder EL. Non-infectious complications of transfusion therapy. Blood Rev. 2001;15:69–83.

Vamvakas EC, Blajchman MA. Universal WBC reduction: the case for and against. Transfusion. 2001;41:691–712.

Answer to question 149: C

Educational objective

To recognize the impact of specimen turbidity on hemoglobin measurement

Critique

The total red cell count, mean platelet volume and mean corpuscular volume are not affected by turbidity. Improperly lysed red cells, leukocytosis, paraproteinemia and hyperlipidemia can artifactually increase the hemoglobin concentration by increasing sample turbidity.

References

Cornbleet J. Spurious results from automated hematology cell analyzers. Lab Med. 1983;14:509–14.

Grimaldi E, Scopacasa F. Evaluation of the Abbott CELL-DYN 4000 hematology analyzer. Am J Clin Pathol. 2000;113:497–505.

Answer to question 150: B

Educational objective

To treat pre-eclampsia

Critique

Pre-eclampsia occurs in 5–10% of all pregnancies and is more common in primigravida African-Americans with diabetes. The syndrome consists of the gradual onset of hypertension, edema and proteinuria during the third trimester. Headache is a common symptom. Laboratory abnormalities include thrombocytopenia (15%), anemia, mild schistocytosis and mild elevation of creatinine, bilirubin and hepatic transaminases. "HELLP" is the constellation of microangiopathic **H**emolytic anemia, **E**levated **L**iver function tests and **L**ow **P**latelet count. The term "HELLP syndrome" is misleading since the constellation of findings is not linked by a common etiology, a predictable course or a plan of management in which the three elements are treated together. However, the constellation identified as HELLP syndrome is often seen in pre-eclampsia. The management of pre-eclampsia is of some urgency and is best performed by lowering the blood pressure with magnesium sulfate. Without treatment, this patient's pre-eclampsia might progress to eclampsia (grand mal seizures not attributable to another cause and associated with pre-eclampsia). The manifestations of HELLP syndrome often resolve with the subsidence of pre-eclampsia. Hematologic intervention is usually not required. The hematologist should be alert to the possibility that causes other than pre-eclampsia may have resulted in thrombocytopenia and anemia and be prepared to intervene after the blood pressure is controlled, particularly if hematologic manifestations worsen after pre-eclampsia resolves. Consideration should be given to less common but serious complications of pregnancy such as TTP–HUS, hepatorenal syndrome or DIC. The hallmarks of TTP–HUS are fragmented red cells (schistocytes) and a high LDH, findings that should prompt consideration of potentially life-saving plasma exchange. Patients with HELLP syndrome who have pre-existing severe or chronic liver disease should be watched carefully for signs of renal failure, a symptom complex known as hepatorenal syndrome. Although quite rare, DIC may first be manifest by HELLP syndrome and pre-eclampsia brought on by complications of pregnancy such as abruptio placenta. DIC with abruptio placenta is more likely in multiparas with chronic hypertension than in previously normotensive primiparas, and is usually associated with vaginal bleeding, lower abdominal pain and signs of fetal distress. If DIC develops, a live birth is highly unlikely, although the pregnancy should be terminated in the hope of saving the mother.

Reference

Hollenberg NK. A comparison of magnesium sulfate and nimodipine for the prevention of eclampsia. Curr Hypertens Rep. 2003;5:288.

Answer to question 151: A

Educational objective

To treat a patient with paroxysmal nocturnal hemoglobinuria complicating aplastic anemia

Critique

This patient has a coexistent paroxysmal nocturnal hemoglobinuria (PNH) and aplastic anemia (AA). The PNH in such patients is often clinically silent (therefore this patient is atypical). It is possible that immune-mediated marrow suppression acts as a selective force for PNH or myelodysplastic syndrome (MDS) clones in AA, although this has not been proven.

The treatment strategy in such patients is to treat them as for AA. The PNH clone *per se* is not an indication for stem cell transplant as the initial treatment. This patient's older age and his mild disease suggest the use of immunosuppression as the initial treatment. If the patient demonstrates evidence of MDS, another clonal disorder in the differential diagnosis, then stem cell transplant might be considered. PNH is associated with an increased risk for intravascular thrombosis, often in unusual sites such as the portal system or the brain. Anticoagulation or thrombolytic therapy is required for treatment of venous thrombosis. Prophylactic anticoagulation (or antiplatelet therapy) can be considered in patients with PNH; however, in patients without a history of thrombosis and in whom bone marrow failure appears to be the predominant problem (as in this patient), it is not usual practice.

Reference

Young NS. The problem of clonality in aplastic anemia: Dr Dameshek's riddle, restated. Blood. 1992;79:1385–92.

Answer to question 152: B

Educational objective

To identify the association of hepatitis C with porphyria cutanea tarda

Critique

This patient presents with blistering skin lesions, has prior intravenous drug and current ethyl alcohol use, all of which are noted with increased frequency in patients with porphyria cutanea tarda (PCT). In fact, many patients with the genetic mutations leading to PCT only become symptomatic when exposed to excessive iron through such risk factors as hepatitis C, ethyl alcohol or hereditary hemochromatosis. This patient should have liver function and hepatitis tests checked. Patients with AIP do not have skin lesions and so testing for urine ALA and PBG as well as red cell PBG levels is not necessary. If hemochromatosis evaluation is to be pursued, genetic testing should first be performed in the patient in order to establish the diagnosis before testing of his children is carried out.

References

Cohen DJ, McKay M. Porphyria cutanea tarda: a clinical review. Compr Ther. 1996;22:175–8.

Fargion S, Fracanzani AL. Prevalence of hepatitis C virus infection in porphyria cutanea tarda. J Hepatol. 2003;39:635–8.

Gisbert JP, Garcia-Buey L, Pajares JM, Moreno-Otero R. Prevalence of hepatitis C virus infection in porphyria cutanea tarda: systematic review and meta-analysis. J Hepatol. 2003;39:620–7.

Answer to question 153: D

Educational objective

To recognize pure red cell aplasia resulting from ABO-mismatched bone marrow transplantation

Critique

As many as 20% of recipients of ABO-incompatible bone marrow will develop pure red cell aplasia because of existing isohemagglutinins in the recipients' plasma. The problem most frequently occurs in an O recipient of type A marrow. The problem results in dependence on RBC transfusions with compatible RBCs, and will usually resolve in 6–12 months. Resolution will be hastened by the development of graft-versus-host disease (GVHD). Plasma exchange with replacement with donor's plasma has been helpful in reducing protracted dependence on red cell transfusions. A recent study showed that ABO-mismatched nonmyeloablative allogeneic transplantation is associated with longer hospitalizations and significantly higher transplant-related mortality, but with a decrease in leukemia relapse or progression.

Neither immunosuppressive drugs nor persistent leukemia will result in selective suppression of red cell precursors as noted on bone marrow examination. Aplastic anemia is not a complication associated with bone marrow transplantation, and would not be manifested by selective red cell aplasia as seen in this patient.

References

Worel N, Greinix H, Schneider B, Kurz M, Rabitsch W, Knobl P, et al. Regeneration of erythropoiesis after related- and unrelated-donor BMT or peripheral blood HPC transplantation: a major ABO mismatch means problems. Transfusion. 2000;40:543–50.

Worel N, Kalhs P, Keil F, Prinz E, Moser K, Schulenburg A, et al. ABO mismatch increases transplant related morbidity and mortality in patients given nonmyeloablative allogeneic HPC transplantation. Transfusion. 2003;43:1153–61.

Answer to question 154: C

Educational objective

To treat cold agglutinin disease in a patient with cardiopulmonary compromise

Critique

This patient presents with weight loss, fever, chills and night sweats suggestive of lymphoma. His laboratory data are consistent with hemolysis, and red cell agglutination is seen on review of the blood smear. In addition, the MCV is markedly elevated, although likely spurious. All of these findings support the diagnosis of cold agglutinin disease. The patient is not responding to blood transfusion and is currently experiencing unstable angina. Plasma exchange therapy through a blood warmer can transiently decrease the IgM antibody titer and potentially lessen the ongoing hemolysis. It should be considered as initial treatment in this case given cardiac compromise and lack of response to transfusion. Cytotoxic therapy is indicated for long-term control when the patient is stabilized. The cytotoxic drug regimen can be tailored to treat an underlying lymphoma if it is subsequently diagnosed. Steroids are usually not effective in idiopathic cold agglutinin disease, although administration is appropriate with the diagnosis of lymphoma. Splenectomy is a treatment for warm autoimmune hemolytic anemia but is usually not effective in cold agglutinin disease. If further blood is to be transfused, it should be given through a blood warmer.

References

Andrzejewski C Jr, Gault E, Briggs M, Silberstein L. Benefit of a 37°C extracorporeal circuit in plasma exchange therapy for selected cases with cold agglutinin disease. J Clin Apheresis. 1988;4:13–7.

Gehrs BC, Freidberg RC. Autoimmune hemolytic anemia. Am J Hematol. 2002;69:258–71.

Answer to question 155: D

Educational objective

To evaluate a patient with possible Philadelphia (Ph) chromosome-negative chronic myeloid leukemia (CML)

Critique

A minority of patients with CML (5–10%) lack the Ph chromosome [have no detectable t(9;22) karyotypic abnormality]. One-third of patients with clinical and laboratory abnormalities typical of CML and who appear to have a normal karyotype actually have the *BCR-ABL* rearrangement. PCR, to identify the fusion gene or the transcript of the fusion gene, or fluorescence *in situ* hybridization (FISH) analysis of interphase nuclei, can diagnose these cases. The clinical presentation with splenomegaly, presence of immature myeloid forms, presence of basophils on the peripheral smear and long-standing leukocytosis make CML or another myeloproliferative disorder likely. Imatinib is effective for Ph-negative *BCR-ABL*-positive CML because the drug acts to block the tyrosine kinase function of the $p210^{BCR\text{-}ABL}$ oncoprotein. She has had elevated WBC count for at least 6 months and basophils on her peripheral smear, making infection unlikely. The LAP score could be helpful but lacks sensitivity and specificity.

Reference

Goldman JM, Melo JV. Chronic myeloid leukemia: advances in biology and new approaches to treatment. N Engl J Med. 2003;349:1451–64.

Answer to question 156: D

Educational objective

To recognize the characteristic features of alkylator-induced myelodysplastic syndrome

Critique

This unfortunate young girl has developed MDS as a result of therapeutic exposure to mutagenic chemotherapeutic agents and radiation. Cases of therapy-induced myeloid malignancies arising in adults and children share similar clinical and biologic features. In this patient, the time of disease onset and MDS presentation are most consistent with alkylator-induced MDS, which is most often associated with monosomy 7. By contrast, patients who develop therapy-related myeloid malignancies after exposure to etoposide typically present with acute leukemia after shorter latency. Cytogenetic analysis of these cases reveals 11q23 translocations, which fuse the *MLL* gene to multiple partner genes. There is no evidence that intensive chemotherapy improves the dismal outcome in patients with therapy-associated MDS. The most appropriate management for this child is to proceed directly to allogeneic stem cell transplantation after a suitable donor is identified.

References

Le Beau MM, Albain KS, Larson RA, Vardiman JW, Davis EM, Blough RR, et al. Clinical and cytogenetic correlations in 63 patients with therapy-related myelodysplastic syndromes and acute nonlymphocytic leukemia: further evidence for characteristic abnormalities of chromosomes 5 and 7. J Clin Oncol. 1986;3:325–45.

Smith SM, Le Beau MM, Huo D, Karrison T, Sobecks RM, Anastasi J, et al. Clinical–cytogenetic associations in 306 patients with therapy-related myelodysplasia and myeloid leukemia: the University of Chicago series. Blood. 2003;102:43–52.

Answer to question 157: A

Educational objective

To recognize the appropriate maintenance therapy for a patient with APL in complete remission

Critique

Although maintenance therapy in AML has generally not been proven effective, this strategy appears to be an important one in patients with APL. Several large randomized studies have now confirmed that maintenance therapy with either ATRA alone or ATRA plus low-dose chemotherapy (usually 6-mercaptopurine and methotrexate) for 1–2 years prolongs remission duration and may contribute to cure. There is no proven indication for arsenic trioxide as maintenance therapy for patients in first remission. Furthermore, although autologous stem cell transplantation may be useful in patients who relapse and then achieve a second complete molecular remission, there is no role for autologous stem cell transplantation in first remission in patients with APL. The latter strategy could be studied for patients at high risk, but no such studies have been carried out to date.

References

Fenaux P, Chastagne C, Chevret S, et al. A randomized comparison of all-*trans* retinoic acid (ATRA) followed by chemotherapy and ATRA + chemotherapy and the role of maintenance therapy in newly diagnosed acute promyelocytic leukemia. The European APL Group. Blood. 1999;94:1192–200.

Sanz MA, Lo Coco FL, Martin G, et al. Definition of relapse risk and the role of non-anthracycline drugs for consolidation in patients with acute promyelocytic leukemia: a joint study by the PETHEMA and GIMEMA cooperative groups. Blood. 2000;96:1247–53.

Tallman MS, Andersen JW, Schiffer CA, et al. All-*trans* retinoic acid in acute promyelocytic leukemia. N Engl J Med. 1997;337:1021–8.

Answer to question 158: D

Educational objective

To recognize the late complication of therapy-related second malignancy in patients treated for Hodgkin disease

Critique

This patient presents 9 years after primary radiation therapy for Hodgkin lymphoma. As patients approach 10 years from treatment they are more likely to die from a secondary malignancy than from recurrent Hodgkin lymphoma. Tumors related to radiation therapy appear in or at the edge of the radiation field and women with radiation to breast tissue are at high risk. Lung cancer and breast cancers in women are the most common second malignancies because of their frequency in the population, despite having lower relative risk. Because of this increased risk, it is recommended that women begin yearly screening mammography within 10 years of undergoing radiation therapy.

Although CT scanning and PET scanning are valuable for monitoring response to therapy, there would be no role for either in this patient at very low risk of relapse. A yearly complete blood count would be reasonable in a patient with previous exposure to alkylating agents because of the risk of subsequent MDS/AML, but would not be necessary in this patient.

Reference

Aisenberg AC. Problems in Hodgkin's disease management. Blood. 1999;93:761.

Answer to question 159: C

Educational objective

To recognize heparin-induced thrombocytopenia

Critique

The patient should be considered to have heparin-induced thrombocytopenia (HIT). If available, serological testing should be submitted for evaluation. The patient's *baseline* platelet count is likely markedly elevated because of his previous splenectomy. A count of 160/μL is thus likely a fall of >50% from baseline. The myocardial infarction and arterial thrombosis are likely both consequences of HIT which initially developed in response to the heparin administered at the time of the angiogram. The prothrombotic condition would have been worsened by heparin received at the time of the PCI. Both heparin and LMWH are likely to worsen the HIT; thus, the treatment of choice is lepirudin. Warfarin should be overlapped with the lepirudin; however, warfarin should not be started until the platelet count is at or above baseline. Although thrombolysis might be used in this setting to treat acute arterial ischemia it should not be used in concert with heparin.

Reference

Hirsh J, Heddle N, Kelton JG. Treatment of heparin-induced thrombocytopenia: a critical review. Arch Intern Med. 2004;164:361–69.

Answer to question 160: D

Educational objective

To recognize the indication for prophylactic platelet transfusion

Critique

The effectiveness of prophylactic platelet transfusion in the prevention of hemorrhage has not been validated through randomized prospective clinical study, but it has become the standard of care to transfuse platelets before a patient has significant bleeding in a number of clinical settings, especially hematologic malignancy. The goal of most prophylactic transfusions is to achieve a sustained increment of the circulating platelet count, because historical data showed that there was an almost linear correlation between platelet count and bleeding once moderate to severe thrombocytopenia developed, and cessation of thrombocytopenic bleeding was seen only when an increment was achieved. Historical triggers of ≥20,000/μL were misadapted from older literature in leukemic patients and should be discarded today. Many of those patients also received aspirin as antipyretic therapy, and in addition the data did not support a single platelet count as a trigger. Some recent studies, including one randomized trial in AML patients, have shown that significant major bleeding is not increased until a platelet of ≤10,000/μL is reached, unless other factors that predispose to hemorrhage are present. These include fever, infection, malnutrition, mucositis, other coagulopathy or concomitant anatomic defects such as gastrointestinal pathology or CNS tumors. However, these studies showed an increase in minor bleeding at this low threshold, and the practice of withholding platelet transfusion until the count is <10,000/μL has not been validated as a completely safe practice. Because of this, the options purposely excluded this 10,000/μL level. In the absence of other risk factors, as in this patient, there appears to be a consensus that a threshold of 15,000/μL is safe and adequate and that triggers at higher levels are unnecessary. Bone marrow transplantation especially may require a higher 'transfusion trigger' in view of the cytokine storm seen post-transplant and the sequelae of high-dose therapy, and some programs use a trigger of ≥15,000/μL for those patients because they commonly have additional risk factors for bleeding. Platelet transfusion to 'cover' invasive procedures is frequently practiced, but there is debate about what a safe target should be for line placement, lumbar puncture, bronchoscopy or colonoscopy. Most surgical procedures can safely occur when the platelet count is >40,000–50,000/μL.

References

Beutler E. Platelet transfusions: the 20,000/μL trigger. Blood. 1993;81:1411–3.

Gaydos LA, Freireich EI, Mantel N. The quantitative relationship between platelet count and hemorrhage in patients with acute leukemia. N Engl J Med. 1962;266:905–9.

Rebulla P, Finazzi G, Marangoni F, Avvisati G, Gugliotta L, Tognoni G, et al. The threshold for prophylactic platelet transfusions in adults with acute myeloid leukemia. N Engl J Med. 1997;337:1870–5.

Answer to question 161: C

Educational objective

To diagnose nodular lymphocyte-predominant Hodgkin disease

Critique

Nodular lymphocyte-predominant Hodgkin disease is a monoclonal B-cell lymphoma. The pattern on lymph node biopsy is either nodular or nodular and diffuse. L and H cells (lymphocytic and/or histiocytic Reed–Sternberg cell variants) are characteristic of this lymphoma. Mediastinal, splenic and bone marrow involvement are infrequent; most patients present with stage I–II disease. The tumor cells are CD20, CD45, BCL6 and surface immunoglobulin positive. EMA is positive in 50% of cases. CD5, CD10, CD15 and CD30 are negative. Follicular lymphomas are typically CD10 positive, mantle cell lymphomas are typically CD5 positive and lymphocyte-rich classic Hodgkin disease Reed–Sternberg cells are CD30 and CD15 positive and negative for CD45.

References

Fan Z, Natkunam Y, Bair E, Tibshirani R, Warnke RA, et al. Characterization of variant patterns of nodular lymphocyte predominant Hodgkin lymphoma with immunohistochemical and clinical correlation. Am J Surg Pathol. 2003;27:1346–56.

Jaffe ES, Harris NL, Stein H, Vardiman JW. WHO Tumours of Haematopoietic and Lymphoid Tissues. Lyon: IARC Press, 2001.

Answer to question 162: A

Educational objective

To recognize the relative risk of thrombophilia in pregnancy

Critique

Acquired thrombophilia associated with antiphospholipid antibodies (aPL) is reported to be the most common thrombophilia associated with recurrent fetal death particularly in the first trimester. However, in the absence of a personal history of VTE and only a single fetal loss, a positive test for aPL would be insufficient evidence to establish a diagnosis in this patient or to institute treatment. In Western populations, the most common hereditary thrombophilia associated with recurrent fetal loss is heterozygosity for factor V Leiden, which is rare in Chinese. Protein C deficiency and antithrombin III deficiency substantially raise the risk of fetal loss but are much rarer than acquired aPL. Heterozygous factor II G20210A and protein S deficiency should also be considered. This patient's family history and single spontaneous abortion do not constitute sufficient evidence to screen for thrombophilia during pregnancy. An extensive battery of tests would be required to rule out thrombophilia. The first trimester is not an ideal time to perform the tests on this patient because the results are often abnormal during pregnancy, making management decisions problematic. For the patient described in this case, the risks of anticoagulation, including bleeding and other complications, exceed the risk of fetal loss related to thrombophilia. The consultant should advise the patient that studies have not been performed that support the institution of antithrombotic prophylaxis in an established pregnancy. A recent controlled trial in patients with an established diagnosis of thrombophilia and at least one episode of fetal loss after the tenth week supported the use of low-molecular-weight heparin prophylaxis.

References

Brenner B. Clinical management of thrombophilia related placental vascular complications. Blood. 2004;103:4003.

Gris JC, Mercier E, Quere I, Lavigne-Lissalde G, Cochery-Nouvellon E, Hoffet M, et al. Low-molecular-weight heparin versus low-dose aspirin in women with one fetal loss and a constitutional thrombophilic disorder. Blood. 2004;103:3695–9.

Answers to question 163: (a) D, (b) C

Educational objective

To recognize myelodysplastic syndrome as a late complication of aplastic anemia and identify a suitable treatment option

Critique

This patient has myelodysplastic syndrome (MDS) as a late complication of severe aplastic anemia. MDS or acute myeloid leukemia (AML) occur as a late complication in as many as 20% of severe aplastic anemia patients treated with antithymocyte globulin (ATG) and cyclosporine immunosuppression. Cytogenetic abnormalities noted in this setting are typical for MDS and include monosomy 7 and trisomy 8 (which can also occur together). These cytogenetic abnormalities are associated with a poor prognosis in MDS. AML-type induction and consolidation chemotherapy is not appropriate at this time as the patient does not have AML. For patients with AML and chromosome 7 or complex cytogenetic abnormalities, standard AML induction and consolidation chemotherapy is associated with long-term survival of <5–10%. Immunosuppression with ATG and cyclosporine could be considered to treat the cytopenia in this patient; however, it is very unlikely that such treatment would eradicate the myelodysplastic clone or be curative in this patient. Stem cell transplant is the only curative option available for patients with MDS. In this patient without a potential sibling donor, matched unrelated donor stem cell transplant offers a reasonable chance of cure. Outcomes with matched unrelated stem cell transplant are best in patients under the age of 20 years. Matched unrelated donor stem cell transplantation is considered for patients as old as 50 years with high-risk MDS or AML. The presence of the monosomy 7 abnormality in this patient's cytogenetic studies suggests that her disease has a high risk of progressing.

The chromosomal abnormalities t(8;21) and inv16 are associated with *de novo* AML and are not typically seen with MDS or AML evolving from aplastic anemia. The t(4;11) abnormality is seen in some cases of acute lymphoblastic leukemia.

Reference

Deeg HJ, Appelbaum FR. Hematopoietic stem cell transplantation in patients with myelodysplastic syndrome. Leuk Res. 2000;24:653–63.

Answer to question 164: A

Educational objective

To recognize parvovirus B19 as a cause of aplastic crisis in patients with chronic hemolytic anemias, and to recognize the potentially chronic nature of parvovirus B19 in HIV-infected patients

Critique

Any insult that results in decreased erythrocyte production will lead to a rapid and significant decrease in the H/H in a patient with chronic hemolysis. Parvovirus B19, the etiology of fifth disease in childhood, will selectively infect red cell precursors, leading to reticulocytopenia and a rapid fall in H/H in patients with sickle cell disease, and is a well-known cause of aplastic crisis in these patients.

A significant portion of adult sickle cell patients have transfusion-transmitted diseases such as HIV-1 and hepatitis C as a result of blood product exposure in the past. Parvovirus B19 infection may become chronic in HIV-infected patients, leading to anemia. Several reports have documented the usefulness of intravenous gammaglobulin therapy in the treatment of parvovirus infection in HIV-infected patients. AZT monotherapy, a frequent cause of anemia, would not be expected to help correct parvovirus-induced anemia. Combination therapy with interferon-α and ribavirin is useful in treating hepatitis C, but would not be expected to have a role in treating parvovirus; in addition, ribavirin results in red cell hemolysis and must be used with great caution in patients with hemolytic disorders. Trimethoprim-sulfamethoxazole has been implicated in bone marrow suppression and would have no beneficial effect on parvovirus. Because adult sickle cell patients have little or no remaining spleen tissue, splenectomy is not a reasonable option.

References

Fuller A, Moaven L, Spelman D, Spicer W, Wraight H, Curtis D, et al. Parvovirus B19 in HIV infection: a treatable cause of anemia. Pathology. 1996;28:277–80.

Koduri PR. Parvovirus B19-related anemia in HIV-infected patients. AIDS Patient Care Stds. 2000;14:7–11.

Mallouh A, Qudah A. Acute splenic sequestration together with aplastic crisis caused by human parvovirus B19 in patients with sickle cell disease. J Pediatr. 1993;122:593–5.

Answer to question 165: A

Educational objective

To recognize the presentation and typical peripheral blood smear findings seen with traumatic hemolysis

Critique

The patient has symptomatic anemia, jaundice and an elevated reticulocyte count, suggesting a hemolytic process. On physical examination, he has a heart murmur over the aortic valve. Echocardiogram confirms a perivalvular leak. Dysfunction of prosthetic heart valves can lead to traumatic hemolysis. The classic red cell morphology on the blood smear is schistocytes. Treatment often requires valve replacement, but iron and erythropoietin can be tried in patients who are poor surgical candidates. Bite cells, resulting from the denaturing of hemoglobin, would be seen in G6PD deficiency or with an unstable hemoglobin, spherocytes in autoimmune hemolytic anemia or hereditary spherocytosis, and stomatocytes with rare inherited hemolytic anemia or in otherwise healthy individuals.

References

Mecozzi G, Milano AD, De Carlo M, Sorrentino F, Pratali S, Nardi C, et al. Intravascular hemolysis in patients with new-generation prosthetic heart valves: a prospective study. J Thorac Cardiovasc Surg. 2002;123:550–6.

Shapira Y, Bairey O, Vatury M, Magen-Nativ H, Prokocimer M, Sagie A. Erythropoietin can obviate the need for repeated heart valve replacement in high-risk patients with severe mechanical hemolytic anemia: case reports and literature review. J Heart Valve Dis. 2001;10:431–5.

Answer to question 166: D

Educational objective

To treat chronic myeloid leukemia (CML) in blast crisis

Critique

This patient presents with CML in myeloid blast crisis. The aim of therapy in this setting is to first re-establish chronic phase or achieve a remission with imatinib or induction chemotherapy, and then to proceed to allogeneic stem cell transplantation if a donor can be identified. Autologous transplantation does not have a role in blast crisis. Patients with myeloid blast crisis treated with conventional induction chemotherapy achieve a second chronic phase in 20–30% of cases; however, relapse inevitably occurs even with intensification. Imatinib, at higher doses (600–800 mg/day), can re-establish chronic phase in a greater proportion of patients than conventional induction chemotherapy, but still usually for only a short duration. Imatinib with or without induction chemotherapy is currently being tested as a bridge to allogeneic transplant. At the present time, a standard approach is to use induction chemotherapy for CML myeloid blast crisis and proceed to allogeneic transplant when feasible.

References

Deininger MW, O'Brien SG, Ford JM, Druker BJ. Practical management of patients with chronic myeloid leukemia receiving imatinib. J Clin Oncol. 2003;21:1637–47.

National Comprehensive Cancer Network (NCCN) Clinical Practice Guidelines in Oncology. Chronic myelogenous leukemia. J Natl Compr Cancer Network: JNCCN. 2003;1:482–500.

Wayne AS, Barrett AJ. Allogeneic hematopoietic stem cell transplantation for myeloproliferative disorders and myelodysplastic syndromes. Hematol Oncol Clin North Am. 2003;17:1175–90.

Answer to question 167: D

Educational objective

To treat an older patient with relapsed AML

Critique

The outcome for adults with AML who relapse after a first remission is poor. The likelihood of successful reinduction with salvage cytotoxic chemotherapy is directly related to the duration of first remission. For patients whose first remission duration is generally more than 1–2 years, reinduction chemotherapy with high-dose cytarabine for those patients not participating in a clinical trial has become a routine approach. There is no evidence that adding additional agents such as daunorubicin or mitoxantrone to cytarabine is useful. The immunoconjugate gemtuzumab ozogamicin has been recently approved for the treatment of older adults in first relapse who are not suitable candidates for cytotoxic chemotherapy. This immunoconjugate contains an anti-CD33 antibody chemically linked to a potent toxin called calicheamicin. The overall remission rate in older adults in first relapse, with a first remission duration >6 months, is approximately 30%. There is no definitive evidence as yet that combining any chemotherapy with gemtuzumab ozogamicin is a useful strategy, but this approach is the subject of current ongoing clinical trials.

References

Estey EH. Treatment of relapsed and refractory acute myelogenous leukemia. Leukemia. 2000;14:476–9.

Karanes C, Kopecky KJ, Head DR, et al. A phase III comparison of high-dose ara-C (Hi-DAC) versus Hi-DAC plus mitoxantrone in the treatment of first relapsed or refractory acute myeloid leukemia. A Southwest Oncology Group Study. Leuk Res. 1999;23:787–94.

Larson RA, Boogaerts M, Estey E, et al. Antibody-targeted chemotherapy of older patients with acute myeloid leukemia in first relapse using Mylotarg (gemtuzumab ozogamicin). Leukemia. 2002;16:1627–36.

Sievers EL, Larson RA, Stadtmauer EA, et al. Efficacy and safety of gemtuzumab ozogamicin in patients with CD33-positive acute myeloid leukemia in first relapse. J Clin Oncol. 2001;19:3244–54.

Answer to question 168: D

Educational objective

To identify the role of bortezomib in relapsed and refractory multiple myeloma

Critique

This patient has relapsed multiple myeloma and requires therapy. High-dose therapy with autologous stem cell rescue has been shown to improve survival in selected patients with myeloma, although many patients relapse, as in this case. The proteosome inhibitor, bortezomib, is indicated for patients with relapsed and refractory multiple myeloma based on response rates of 35% in heavily pretreated patients. Treatment with melphalan and prednisone would not be expected to have a significant impact on refractory disease in this case, and retreatment with high-dose therapy would not be an option because of excess toxicity. Continuing treatment with a bisphosphonate is important for patients with lytic lesions, but would not affect the progression of his disease. Palliative care would also be an option, particularly for a patient with a poor performance status or a desire to avoid further cytotoxic therapy.

Reference

Richardson P, Barlogie B, Berenson J, Singhal S, Jagannath S, Irwin D, et al. A phase 2 study of bortezomib in relapsed, refractory myeloma. N Engl J Med. 2003;348:2609–17.

Answer to question 169: D

Educational objective

To provide perioperative care for a patient taking warfarin

Critique

This patient has a number of high-risk features for stroke when warfarin is discontinued. Although simple discontinuation of warfarin may be an acceptable treatment in this case, it might place the patient at risk of avoidable stroke, and if it is stopped 72 h prior to the procedure there is a high risk of a persistent coagulopathy at the time of surgery. Admission to hospital for intravenous unfractionated heparin remains an acceptable treatment; however, admission to receive low-dose unfractionated heparin cannot be justified as this treatment can be safely and effectively delivered at home. Although use of prophylactic dose enoxaparin may be acceptable for prevention of arterial thromboembolism, the usual prophylactic dose is 30 mg twice daily. In some centers warfarin is not withheld for orthopedic surgery; rather the target INR is reduced and the patient will go to surgery with an INR of 1.5–2.0. This strategy is likely safe; however, it is not well validated. Even in centers that use this approach, the INR is rarely >2.0 at the time of the procedure.

Reference

Douketis JD. Perioperative anticoagulation management in patients who are receiving oral anticoagulant therapy: a practical guide for clinicians [Comment]. Thromb Res. 2002;108:3–13.

Answer to question 170: E

Educational objective

To recognize post-transfusion circulatory overload in an infant

Critique

This infant has many of the signs associated with circulatory overload following transfusion. The small body size of newborns and infants correlates with a smaller total blood volume and makes them particularly susceptible to this type of reaction. The elderly are also likely to be at risk for these reactions, as they lose vascular compliance and develop cardiopulmonary impairment. Transfusion therapy in pediatrics is frequently limited by the small blood volume, making dose calculations on the basis of volume rather than product content common. In the absence of anuria, most infants can tolerate 10–15 mL/kg without concern for volume overload. When larger deficits need replacement, frequent small transfusions or exchange transfusion can be employed. The volume of a unit of packed cells, when collected in the highly prevalent additive solutions now used for blood preservation, is approximately 350 mL. This is between three or four times greater than the usual dose of replacement red cells for an infant. Bacterial contamination is rarely a problem with red cell transfusion in view of the refrigerated storage. Atopy is usually not manifest until the second or third year of life, and signs of anaphylaxis were not present. No evidence in support of blood incompatibility or hemolysis was evident, and most packed cell units contain such little residual plasma that the small amount of anti-A in a group O unit is insignificant. This is especially true for packed cells collected in AS-1 rather than CPDA-1, because the higher volume of the storage medium does not require residual anticoagulated plasma to maintain cell viability. Infants are limited in their ability to become alloimmunized, and the father is not at risk for prior alloimmunization, making leukoagglutinin reactions unlikely.

References

Goodstein MH, Locke RG, Wlodarczyk D, Goldsmith LS, Rubenstein SD, Herman JH. Comparison of two preservation solutions for erythrocyte transfusions in newborn infants. J Pediatr. 1993;123:783–8.

Hume H, Bard H. Small volume red blood cell transfusions for neonatal patients. Transfus Med Rev. 1995;9:187–99.

Paul DA, Leef KH, Locke RG, Stefano JL. Transfusion volume in infants with very low birth weight: a randomized trial of 10 versus 20 mL/kg. J Pediatr Hematol Oncol. 2002;24:43–6.

Answer to question 171: C

Educational objective

To recognize the typical cytogenetic abnormality of acute promyelocytic leukemia

Critique

Hypogranular acute promyelocytic leukemia (APL) is often confused with acute monocytic leukemia because of the nuclear shape. The azurophilic granules in hypogranular APL are submicroscopic. In general, patients with hypogranular APL have a high leukocyte count. Disseminated intravascular coagulation is common in both the hyper- and hypogranular forms. The t(15;17)(q22;q12) is the typical cytogenetic abnormality seen in APL.

The t(1;22) is seen in young children with acute megakaryoblastic leukemia; the prognosis is poor. The t(8;21)(q22;q22) is seen predominantly in acute myeloid leukemia with maturation; the prognosis is good. The t(8;16)(p11;p13) is seen in acute monoblastic and acute monocytic leukemia associated with hemophagocytosis.

References

Parmar S, Tallman MS. Acute promyelocytic leukemia: a review. Exp Opin Pharmacother. 2003;4:1379–92.

Redner RL. Variations on a theme: the alternate translocations in APL. Leukemia. 2002;16:1927–32.

Answer to question 172: D

Educational objective

To manage mild thrombocytopenia

Critique

Continuation of periodic platelet counts is the most appropriate approach because the thrombocytopenia is chronic, mild and relatively asymptomatic. The 2-year chronicity makes nonprogressive disease a possibility, although the recent decline in the platelet count bears watching. Diseases with insidious onset, such as myelodysplastic syndrome and Gaucher's disease, should be considered. The relatively brief bleeding from shaving cuts and two unexplained bruises do not constitute a significant bleeding risk. Post-traumatic bleeding or epistaxis lasting over 15 min, ecchymoses, hematomas and petechiae would be of greater concern. Antibody studies would not change the approach to management even if they were positive. CT scans of the chest and abdomen to rule out a malignant disease, such as lymphoma, are not justified by the information provided. Similarly, a bone marrow examination would not influence management at this time because intervention is based on clinical findings, although isolated thrombocytopenia as a manifestation of myelodysplastic syndrome is a consideration, because management would not be affected. Mild chronic thrombocytopenia, sometimes a consequence of ITP, may persist for years and does not require intervention if the platelet count is >70,000/μL.

Reference

George JN. Idiopathic thrombocytopenic purpura: current issues for pathogenesis, diagnosis, and management in children and adults. Curr Hematol Rep. 2003;2:381.

Answer to question 173: D

Educational objective

To manage persistent bleeding in a newborn

Critique

Although the history is suggestive of an inherited bleeding disorder, a definitive diagnosis has not been established. A comprehensive laboratory evaluation is indicated and a plasma sample should be immediately obtained from the patient for this purpose. It may take days to establish the precise diagnosis of the hemorrhagic disorder, but immediate intervention is needed to stop the bleeding. Management of a bleeding disorder of unknown or unconfirmed etiology is best accomplished with fresh frozen plasma (FFP). FFP is also the specific therapy for factor V and XI deficiency as no individual factor preparation is available for these deficiencies. A dose of 10 mL/kg FFP will raise plasma coagulation factors by approximately 20%, sufficient for hemostasis. However, caution is appropriate. Administration of FFP to a neonate may increase the risk of thrombosis because of a relative deficiency of proteins involved in fibrinolysis. Cryoprecipitate is an excellent concentrated source of factor VIII, factor XIII, von Willebrand factor and fibrinogen but deficient in other plasma factors. Recombinant factor VIII replaces only a single factor and is the therapy of choice only for patients with a confirmed diagnosis of hemophilia A. Recombinant factor VIII lacks von Willebrand factor and is inappropriate for the treatment of von Willebrand disease, which might also cause neonatal bleeding. Although direct pressure could be applied, it is not likely to be the most effective management if bleeding has continued for 2 h.

Reference

Muntean W. Fresh frozen plasma in the pediatric age group and in congenital coagulation factor deficiency. Thromb Res. 2002;1007:S29.

Answer to question 174: D

Educational objective

To identify utility of CD34 analysis in stem cell transplantation

Critique

Stem cells demonstrate the two features of self-renewal and pluripotency. They are probably the cells that reconstitute long-term hematopoiesis in transplantation. Progenitors on the other hand demonstrate the three features of irreversible lineage commitment, limited proliferative capacity and no capacity for self-renewal. They probably confer some short-term hematopoietic recovery after stem cell transplant.

The CD34 glycoprotein is expressed on the surface of approximately 1–4% of low-density marrow mononuclear cells. The CD34$^+$ fraction includes most of the progenitor cells identified by short-term colony assays and long-term culture-initiating cells (LTC-ICs) that are able to generate progenitors or to form tight clusters of blast cells that resemble cobblestone areas (cobblestone area-forming cells [CAFCs]) for at least 5 weeks in long-term bone marrow culture (probably stem cells). To date, several groups have shown that human CD34$^+$ cells contain the overwhelming majority of stem cells capable of fully reconstituting the lymphohematopoietic system in humans after myeloablative chemotherapy and radiation therapy. A small population of CD34$^-$, side population-positive (SP$^+$) stem cells have been identified. Their role in clinical transplantation is unknown at this time. For the above reasons, flow cytometric analysis of peripheral mononuclear cells for CD34 expression can guide the timing of apheresis collection and indicate the adequacy of stem collection for transplant.

Reference

Lanza F, Campioni D, Moretti S et al. CD34 (+) cell subsets and long-term culture colony-forming cells evaluated on both autologous and normal bone marrow stroma predict long-term hematopoietic engraftment in patients undergoing autologous peripheral blood stem cell transplantation. Exp Hematol. 2001;29:1484–93.

Answer to question 175: C

Educational objective

To recognize the laboratory and peripheral blood smear findings associated with hemolysis after infection with *Mycoplasma pneumoniae*

Critique

This patient presents with laboratory data and clinical sequelae consistent with hemolysis associated with an *M. pneumoniae* infection. Although rare, cold agglutinin-induced hemolysis has been described upon recovery of respiratory symptoms. The etiology is caused by complement fixing IgM antibodies which are directed against the red cell antigen I. The typical blood smear finding is red cell agglutination. The markedly elevated MCV is spurious because of the red cell agglutination. With warming of the specimen an accurate MCV may be obtained. An IgG antibody is characteristic of warm autoantibody-induced hemolytic anemia. Typically, these IgG antibodies do not fix complement or do so only weakly. Spherocytes are typically seen on the blood smear in warm autoantibody-induced hemolysis as the IgG-coated red blood cell membrane is removed by macrophages, which leads to a more spherical-shaped red blood cell.

References

Daxbock F, Zedtwitz-Liebenstein K, Burgmann H, Graninger W. Severe hemolytic anemia and excessive leukocytosis masking mycoplasma pneumonia. Ann Hematol. 2001;80:180–2.

Feizi T. Cold agglutinins, the direct Coombs' test and serum immunoglobulins in *Mycoplasma pneumoniae* infection. Ann NY Acad Sci. 1967;143:801–12.

Answer to question 176: D

Educational objective

To recognize the specific myeloid leukemia that affects children with Down syndrome

Critique

Children with Down syndrome may have dysregulation of hematopoiesis in the newborn period. Often this takes the form of a transient myeloproliferative disorder (TMPD) characterized by anemia, thrombopenia and leukocytosis with an excess of blasts in the blood and marrow. The blasts have an M7 phenotype with a mutation in the *GATA1* gene. The disease resolves without treatment in most individuals, although fatal hepatic fibrosis may occur. Approximately 20% of patients with TMPD develop megakaryocytic leukemia by age 3 years. These leukemias have the same *GATA1* mutations that were present at the time of the TMPD. Interestingly, *GATA1* mutations are not seen in Down syndrome patients with other subtypes of AML or in non-Down syndrome patients with M7 or other subtypes of AML. B-precursor ALL, Burkitt leukemia and acute promyelocytic leukemia (M3) are much less frequent in children with Down syndrome, especially under age 3 years. Children with Down syndrome also have an increased incidence of ALL. However, ALL is not usually preceded by TMPD and *GATA*1 mutations are not usually present.

References

Hitzler JK, Cheung J, Scherer SW, Zipursky A. *GATA1* mutations in transient leukemia and acute megakaryoblastic leukemia of Down syndrome. Blood. 2003;101:4301–4.

Mundschau G, Gurbuxani S, Gamis AS, Greene ME, Arceci RJ, Crispino JD. Mutagenesis of *GATA1* is an initiating event in Down syndrome leukemogenesis. Blood. 2003;101:4298–300.

Answer to question 177: B

Educational objective

To identify a patient with amyloidosis

Critique

This patient has a monoclonal protein, hepatomegaly and nephrotic syndrome. This is suspicious for amyloidosis, which occurs more often with lambda monoclonal proteins. Each of the tissue biopsies could provide evidence of amyloid deposition, but the renal biopsy would differentiate between amyloid and light-chain deposition disease. The diagnosis is confirmed by the presence of apple-green birefringence on polarized light examination of the tissue biopsy stained with Congo red. Bone marrow or liver biopsy can be useful for the diagnosis of amyloidosis, but in the presence of renal failure would not address the cause for the renal insufficiency. Plasma exchange is not effective in amyloidosis. Erythropoietin injections would be reasonable to improve the hemoglobin if a diagnosis of amyloidosis is made.

Reference

Pozzi C, Locatelli F. Kidney and liver involvement in monoclonal light chain disorders. Semin Nephrol. 2002;22:319–30.

Answer to question 178: A

Educational objective

To prevent transfusion-related CMV infection

Critique

Leukocyte reduction has the potential to produce many improvements in blood transfusion safety. Reduction of HLA alloimmunization and a decrease in the incidence of febrile nonhemolytic transfusion reactions have been shown to arise from leukocyte reduction. However, the infant immune system is rarely capable of mounting the same alloimmune response seen in older children and adults. While an immunomodulatory effect of transfusion has been postulated, often attributed to the allogeneic leukocytes in blood products, leading to increased risk of cancer recurrence and nosocomial infection, definitive proof of this effect remains elusive. This infant's mother is HIV-positive and hence the infant may also be infected, and premature infants may have an increased risk of acquiring transfusion-induced GVHD because their immune system is incapable of preventing the donor leukocyte response. However, leukocyte reduction has not been validated as an effective method of transfusion-induced GVHD prophylaxis and irradiation of cellular blood components remains the sole licensed and accepted method to prevent GVHD. For over 20 years, CMV infection has been a concern for premature infants, especially those born to seronegative mothers who may not have acquired passive immunity. Neonatal hepatitis, pneumonitis, gastroenteritis and marrow failure can be seen in premature infants suffering from systemic CMV infection. CMV is a cell-borne virus and transmission by plasma has not been demonstrated. Relatively inefficient methods of leukocyte removal, such as frozen, washed red cells and buffy coat removal, were shown to be effective at preventing CMV transmission through transfusion in the newborn before being supplanted by serologic screening of donors and the use of CMV seronegative units. The newer filtration technology that can achieve 3 and even 4 log removal of leukocytes has clearly been validated as a safe CMV preventive measure in the newborn, and is an equally effective method to prevent transfusion-acquired CMV infection.

References

Hume H, Bard H. Small volume red blood cell transfusions for neonatal patients. Transfus Med Rev. 1995;9:187–99.

Seftel MD, Growe GH, Petraszko T, Benny WB, Le A, Lee CY, et al. Universal prestorage leukoreduction in Canada decreases platelet alloimmunization and refractoriness. Blood. 2004;103:333–9.

Visconti MR, Pennington J, Garner SF, Allain JP, Williamson LM. Assessment of removal of human cytomegalovirus from blood components by leukocyte depletion filters using real-time quantitative PCR. Blood. 2004;103:1137–9.

Answer to question 179: B

Educational objective

To prescribe preoperative transfusion therapy for a patient with sickle cell anemia

Critique

Preoperative transfusion therapy has been credited with improved morbidity and mortality in patients with sickle cell disease undergoing surgical procedures. However, few prospective randomized trials have been performed to provide objective supportive evidence. In a multicenter national cooperative trial, an intensive preoperative transfusion regimen designed to lower the hemoglobin S level below 30% was found to be no more effective than a more conservative transfusion regimen designed to increase the hemoglobin level to 10 g/dL. A simple transfusion of approximately 10 mL/kg will raise the hemoglobin level by 2–3 g/dL. Evidence does not support the use of exchange transfusion, hydroxyurea therapy or maintenance of oxygen saturation >95%.

References

Ohene-Frempong K. Indications for red cell transfusion in sickle cell disease. Semin Hematol. 2001;38:5.

Riddington C, Williamson L. Preoperative blood transfusions for sickle cell disease. Cochrane Database Syst Rev. 2001:3:CD003149.

Answer to question 180: E

Educational objective

To recognize the clinical and laboratory findings of pyruvate kinase deficiency

Critique

This patient has a congenital nonspherocytic hemolytic

anemia. Pyruvate kinase deficiency is the most common enzymopathy of the Embden–Meyerhof pathway and the characteristic red cell abnormality on the peripheral smear is the echinocyte. Following splenectomy, the reticulocyte count may remain substantially elevated even with improvement in anemia. Patients often exhibit reasonable exercise tolerance. The peripheral blood smear in pyrimidine-5′-nucleotidase deficiency shows prominent basophilic stippling of red cells. Hemoglobin electrophoresis would be useful to assess for a hemoglobinopathy if sickle cells or target cells were seen on blood smear or if an unstable or variant hemoglobin was suspected. Bite cells would be indicative of G6PD deficiency or an unstable hemoglobin. A DAT would be useful to evaluate for warm autoimmune hemolytic anemia if spherocytes were seen and a lifelong history of anemia was not given.

References

Fujii H, Miwa S. Other erythrocyte enzyme deficiencies associated with non-haematological symptoms: phosphoglycerate kinase and phosphofructokinase deficiency. Best Pract Res Clin Haematol. 2000;13:141–8.

Tanaka KR, Paglia DE. Pyruvate kinase deficiency. Semin Hematol. 1971;8:367–96.

Valentine WN, Tanaka KR, Paglia DE. Hemolytic anemias and erythrocyte enzymopathies. Ann Intern Med. 1985;103:245–57.

Answer to question 181: B

Educational objective

To treat a child with granulocytic sarcoma (chloroma)

Critique

Chloromas may develop prior to, concomitant with, or after diagnosis of AML. They are a nodular collection of myeloblasts. Up to 10% of patients with AML may develop a chloroma at some time during their disease. Most chloromas respond completely to systemic chemotherapy. Irradiation can be reserved for patients with an incomplete response to chemotherapy or those in whom the chloroma is causing significant dysfunction in a critical organ.

References

Dusenbery K, Arthur D, Howells W, et al. Granulocytic sarcomas (chloromas) in pediatric patients with newly diagnosed acute myeloid leukemia. Proc Am Soc Clin Oncol. 1996;15:369.

Shome DK, Gupta NK, Prajapati N, et al. Orbital granulocytic sarcomas (myeloid sarcomas) in acute nonlymphocytic leukemia. Cancer. 1992;70:2298–301.

Answer to question 182: E

Educational objective

To manage monoclonal gammopathy of undetermined significance

Critique

This patient has a monoclonal gammopathy of undetermined significance (MGUS). The incidence of MGUS has been estimated to be approximately 1% of patients >50 years and up to 3% of patients >70 years. Approximately 25% of MGUS patients will eventually develop a lymphoproliferative disorder, so follow-up is warranted. There are no laboratory findings that predict progression, and so it is usually recommended that patients have periodic evaluations with CBC, chemistry, serum protein electrophoresis (SPEP) and skeletal survey. Because approximately two-thirds of patients will never develop a malignant disorder, the use of chemotherapy for an MGUS is not warranted.

Reference

Kyle RA, Rajkumar SV. Monoclonal gammopathies of undetermined significance: a review. Immunol Rev. 2003;194:112–39.

Answer to question 183: B

Educational objective

To recognize the causes of prolonged bleeding in the first year of life

Critique

Factor deficiency bleeding in infancy is often characterized by prolonged oozing from venipuncture, frenulum (oral) bleeds and bleeding from the umbilical cord, and unexplained large hematomas from intramuscular injections. Additionally, there can be associated intracranial hemorrhage and excessive surgical bleeding. It is rare to have joint hemorrhage in the first year of life. When factor deficiency bleeding is suspected, hemophilia should be considered. Screening testing for an inherited bleeding disorder is important (CBC, PT, APTT and fibrinogen) and in this case would rule against moderate to severe hemophilia. von Willebrand disease (VWD) does not usually present with prolonged or delayed bleeding unless the factor VIII level is low and this would have been detected with a prolonged APTT. The 5 M urea solubility test is helpful to screen for severe (homozygous, <2%) factor XIII deficiency, but this disorder is characterized by prompt dissolution of the patient's clot in contrast to the laboratory results noted here. Heterozygous factor XIII deficiency usually does not cause bleeding. No inherited bleeding condition exists with TPA excess, the only such deficiency is of TPA's inhibitor (plasminogen activator inhibitor [PAI-1]). Therefore the correct answer can only be homozygous antiplasmin deficiency, a rare disorder characterized by levels of 0.01–0.15 U/mL, which usually causes a shortened euglobulin lysis time (ELT) (typically <1 h). Treatment of antiplasmin deficiency is usually with antifibrinolytic agents such as aminocaproic acid and occasionally with plasma.

References

Hathaway WE. Factor XIII, α_2-antiplasmin and plasminogen activator inhibitor-1 deficiencies. In: Goodnight SH, Hathaway WE, eds. Disorders of Hemostasis and Thrombosis: a Clinical Guide. New York: McGraw-Hill, 2001:184–91.

Saito H. α_2-Plasmin inhibitor and its deficiency states. J Lab Clin Med. 1988;112:671.

Answer to question 184: B

Educational objective

To provide postoperative prophylaxis for venous thromboembolism

Critique

There are no methodologically rigorous data to guide care in this case. The patient is likely at high risk of recurrent venous thromboembolism (VTE) and so not administering prophylaxis is potentially dangerous. Hospitalization and therapeutic dose unfractionated heparin throughout the course of immobilization is likely overly aggressive and might be associated with osteoporosis. Similarly, all studies of extended duration LMWH have used prophylactic rather than therapeutic doses of LMWH. A recent study has confirmed that therapeutic dose warfarin administered after major orthopedic surgery reduces the risk of symptomatic VTE. Although the patient in this scenario is to undergo different surgery from this patient, enrolled in this trial, the risks of thrombosis in this patient, and those included in the study, are likely to be similar.

References

Crowther MA, Kelton JG. Congenital thrombophilic states associated with venous thrombosis: a qualitative overview and proposed classification system. Ann Intern Med. 2003;138:128–34.

Prandoni P, Bruchi O, Sabbion P, Tanduo C, Scudeller A, Sardella C, et al. Prolonged thromboprophylaxis with oral anticoagulants after total hip arthroplasty, a prospective controlled randomized study. Arch Intern Med. 2002;162:1966–71.

Answer to question 185: B

Educational objective

To recognize that severe hemolytic anemia may occur secondary to hereditary elliptocytosis in African-American neonates

Critique

Hereditary elliptocytosis is the most common intrinsic erythrocyte defect causing hemolysis in black neonates and young infants. The peripheral blood smear resembles that of hereditary pyropoikilocytosis, in that numerous tiny and irregularly shaped teardrop- and oval-shaped cells are noted in addition to the 'classic' elliptocytes. The MCV is often reduced. During the initial weeks of life the anemia improves or resolves, and by 1–2 years of age the morphology is that of typical hereditary elliptocytosis. One parent usually demonstrates elliptocytosis as well. Because of high fetal hemoglobin concentration in the neonate, sickle cell anemia does not cause hemolysis. G6PD deficiency would not cause clinical problems in a term infant, especially female. Neither α nor β thalassemia would present in this manner.

References

Austin RF, Desforges J. Hereditary elliptocytosis: an unusual presentation of hemolysis in the newborn associated with transient morphologic abnormalities. Pediatrics. 1969;44:196–200.

Carpentieri U, Gustavson LP, Haggard ME. Pyknocytosis in a neonate: an unusual presentation of hereditary elliptocytosis. Clin Pediatr. 1977;16:76–8.

Gallagher PG. Update on the clinical spectrum and genetics of red blood cell membrane disorders. Curr Hematol Rep. 2004;3:85–91.

Answer to question 186: D

Educational objective

To recognize the optimal treatment of children with AML

Critique

Bone marrow transplantation from a closely matched sibling (not an identical twin) donor provides the best event-free survival and overall survival for children with AML who are in complete remission after induction chemotherapy. This appears to hold for all age, WBC and cytogenetic risk groups. For patients without a closely matched sibling donor, chemotherapy is the standard of care. Autologous transplantation does not improve outcomes in children. Patients at higher risk of treatment failure (prior myelodysplasia, therapy-related leukemia, very high WBC, *FLT-3* internal tandem duplications) may be considered for unrelated donor stem cell transplantation (UDSCT) if a matched sibling donor is not available. However, the benefit of UDSCT is not established in this setting.

Reference

Woods WG, Neudorf Gold S, et al. A comparison of allogeneic bone marrow transplantation, autologous bone marrow transplantation, and aggressive chemotherapy in children with acute myeloid leukemia in remission: a report from the Children's Cancer Group. Blood. 2001;97:56–662.

Answer to question 187: B

Educational objective

To manage relapsed Hodgkin lymphoma

Critique

Treatment of patients with relapsed Hodgkin lymphoma depends on the initial treatment modality and duration of remission. For patients who recur after radiation therapy for localized disease, excellent long-term survival can be achieved with standard chemotherapy. For those patients who recur after chemotherapy, the duration of remission is an important consideration. If the initial remission is >12 months, standard dose chemotherapy can achieve long-term disease-free survival in up to 25% of patients. Patients with primary refractory disease or who relapse within 1 year of treatment are much less likely to benefit from standard dose chemotherapy. As such, the majority of patients relapsing after primary chemotherapy should be referred for high-dose chemotherapy and autologous stem cell transplantation.

References

Connors JM. Treatment of refractory or relapsed Hodgkin's lymphoma. Hematology. 2003;238–47.

Yuen AR, Rosenberg SA, Hoppe RT, Halpern JD, Horning SJ. Comparison between conventional salvage therapy and high-dose therapy with autografting for recurrent or refractory Hodgkin's disease. Blood. 1997;89:814.

Answer to question 188: C

Educational objective

To diagnose a lupus anticoagulant

Critique

This case is a classic description of a lupus anticoagulant in children. These antibodies are usually of no clinical significance in the pediatric population and are usually related to infection or antibiotic use. They do not cause bleeding and are rarely associated with thrombosis. The patient and family history provide important clues as to whether a laboratory abnormality is the result of a bleeding disorder and, in this case, both are not suggestive of a bleeding disorder. The prolonged APTT is appropriately treated with 1 : 1 mixing with normal plasma and lack of correction suggests that an inhibitor is present. One could utilize other phospholipid-sensitive screening tests (such as the dilute Russell Viper Venom test or lupus-sensitive APTT) to corroborate this finding but the best confirmatory test would be to demonstrate that the inhibitory activity is neutralized by excessive phospholipids by utilizing either platelet extract or synthetic phospholipids.

References

Hathaway WE. Activated partial thromboplastin time and minor coagulopathies. Am J Clin Pathol. 1979;71:22.

Triplett DA. Annotation: laboratory identification of the lupus anticoagulant. Br J Haematol. 1989;72:139.

Triplett DA. Lupus anticoagulants: diagnosis and management. Curr Hematol Rep. 2003;2:271–2.

Answer to question 189: A

Educational objective

To manage hemolytic uremic syndrome in a child

Critique

This patient fulfills the diagnostic criteria of hemolytic uremic syndrome (HUS), which includes the triad of microangiopathic hemolytic anemia, thrombocytopenia and renal insufficiency. The Shiga toxin-producing *Escherichia coli* strains, such as *E. coli* 0157:H7, are major worldwide pathogens capable of producing a diarrheal illness that can progress to HUS. Although many children with hemorrhagic colitis develop coagulation abnormalities, only a few develop full-blown HUS. No specific interventions have been shown to be effective for HUS in children. Standard supportive care includes hospitalization followed by intravenous fluid and electrolyte management. If indicated, transfusion for anemia and dialysis for renal failure should be added. Even with appropriate supportive care, death or permanent end-stage renal disease has been reported in 10–15% of patients. The clinical triad associated with HUS results from toxin-mediated damage to the vascular endothelium, subsequent activation of the coagulation cascade, thrombotic microangiopathy and glomerular damage. To confirm the diagnosis of HUS, it is appropriate to perform a stool culture to identify enterohemorrhagic *E. coli* (*E. coli* 0157:H7) or other verotoxin (Shiga-like toxin)-producing bacteria. Antibacterial therapy is of no proven benefit in this setting. Fresh frozen plasma or plasmapheresis is not of proven value in children with HUS, although it is appropriate therapy for adults with TTP. Antiplatelet therapy with aspirin and dipyridamole has no established role in the treatment of HUS, even though it is known that platelets form small vessel microthrombi in patients with this disorder.

References

Andreoli SP, Trachtman H, Acheson DWK, Siegler RL, Obrig TG. Hemolytic uremic syndrome: epidemiology, pathophysiology and therapy. Pediatr Nephrol. 2002;17:293–8.

Garg AX, Suri RS, Barrowman N, Rehman F, Matsell D, Rosas-Arellano MP et al. Long-term renal prognosis of diarrheal-associated hemolytic uremic syndrome. JAMA. 2003;290:1360–70.

Trachtman H, Cnaan A, Christen E, Gibbs K, Zhao S, Acheson DW et al. Effect of an oral shiga toxin-binding agent on diarrheal-associated hemolytic uremic syndrome in children. JAMA. 2003;290:1337–44.

Siegler RL. Postdiarrheal shiga toxin-mediated hemolytic uremic syndrome. JAMA. 2003;290:1379–81.

Answer to question 190: A

Educational objective

To manage acute long bone infarction in a patient with sickle cell disease

Critique

Osteomyelitis is more common in sickle cell disease than in normal hosts. Salmonella and other gram-negative enteric organisms are seen more commonly in patients with sickle cell disease, but staphylococci remain a common cause of osteomyelitis. However, acute long-bone infarction, often accompanying vaso-occlusive pain at other sites, remains a far more common cause of bone pain in sickle cell patients. In the absence of high fever, extreme toxicity and leukocytosis with immature forms on the blood film, a conservative management approach can be undertaken. Infarction of cortical bone, as well as bone marrow infarction, can be managed with analgesics and fluids. Antibiotics, splinting and orthopedic consultation are not necessary at this time. In this case the patient's swelling and pain resolved over the next 3–4 days.

References

Epps CH, Bryant DD, Coles MJM, Castro O. Osteomyelitis in patients who have sickle-cell disease. J Bone Joint Surg. 1991;73:1281–894.

Keeley K, Buchanan GR. Acute infarction of long bones in children with sickle cell anemia. J Pediatr. 1982;101:170–5.

Answer to question 191: E

Educational objective

To treat relapsed AML in a child

Critique

Patients who relapse during treatment or shortly after completing treatment of AML have a poor prognosis. Although a second remission may be induced, <10% achieve long-term disease-free survival. Allogeneic stem cell transplantation using a closely matched related or unrelated donor may cure 25–35% of patients in this setting. The optimal transplant regimen is constantly changing. Children without a closely matched donor are candidates for less established forms of transplantation (haplo-identical and nonmyeloablative transplants) or other experimental treatments.

Reference

Webb DK, Wheatley K, Harrison G, et al. Outcome for children with relapsed acute myeloid leukemia following initial therapy in the Medical Research Council (MRC) AML 10 trial. MRC Childhood Leukemia Working Party. Leukemia. 1999;13:25–31.

Answer to question 192: A

Educational objective

To treat early-stage non-Hodgkin lymphoma in a child

Critique

Therapy of non-Hodgkin lymphoma in children depends upon the stage, location and pathology of the tumor. This patient has a localized (stage I) tumor. Ninety percent of children with a stage I/II Burkitt or large cell lymphoma can be cured with 9 weeks of CHOP chemotherapy. Local irradiation is not necessary. Intrathecal medication is used only for patients at higher risk of developing CNS involvement (those with head and neck tumors). Patients with stage I/II lymphoblastic non-Hodgkin lymphoma require longer treatment.

References

Link MP, Shuster JJ, Donaldson SS, Berard CW, Murphy SB. Treatment of children and young adults with early-stage non-Hodgkin lymphoma. N Engl J Med. 1997;337:1259–66.

Sandlund JT, Downing JR, Crist WM. Non-Hodgkin's lymphoma in childhood. N Engl J Med. 1996;334:1238–48.

Answer to question 193: D

Educational objective

To diagnose vitamin K deficiency

Critique

There are several causes for vitamin K deficiency during infancy. Early presentation (within 24 h of birth) is usually related to maternal drugs such as warfarin, anticonvulsants (e.g. dilantin) and antituberculosis medication. Classic presentation during the first week of life can also be related to maternal medication as well as lack of vitamin K administration at birth or idiopathic causes. Finally, as in this case, delayed presentation or late vitamin K deficiency can be related to breast feeding along with a lack of vitamin K at birth and concomitant diarrheal illness which limits vitamin K absorption. Additionally, malabsorption syndromes in pediatrics (e.g. cystic fibrosis, biliary atresia or neonatal hepatitis) can also cause late-onset vitamin K deficiency.

References

American Academy of Pediatrics. Vitamin K *ad hoc* task force: controversies concerning vitamin K and the newborn. Pediatrics. 1993;91:1001.

Zipursky A. Prevention of vitamin K deficiency bleeding in newborns: review. Br J Haematol. 1999;104:430.

Answer to question 194: B

Educational objective

To recognize α thalassemia trait

Critique

α Thalassemia trait, in which one of the two α globin genes on each chromosome 16 has been deleted, occurs in 2–3% of African-Americans. It is a diagnosis of exclusion in patients with microcytosis, with or without mild anemia, in whom iron deficiency and β thalassemia have been ruled out. The former diagnosis would be unlikely in an infant whose diet has been normal, and the normal hemoglobin A_2 level excludes the latter. There is no ongoing inflammatory condition, and the MCV is too low to make the anemia of chronic inflammation a likely consideration. Fetal hemoglobin is nonspecifically elevated in any infant with anemia. Neonates with α thalassemia will exhibit an elevation in hemoglobin Bart's (a tetramer of γ chains) on their newborn hemoglobin screen. Documentation of this finding would have confirmed the diagnosis.

Reference

Weatherall DJ. The thalassemias. In: Beutler E, Lichtman MA, Coller BS, Kipps TJ, Seligsohn U, eds. Williams Hematology, 6th edn. New York: McGraw-Hill, 2001:547–80.

Answer to question 195: E

Educational objective

To recognize the long-term effects of treatment for Hodgkin lymphoma in children

Critique

Children respond similarly to adults with the same stage and histology of Hodgkin lymphoma. However, children appear to be at higher risk for many complications of treatment because of their ongoing growth and development and a longer expected life span if they are cured. For example, the risk of leukemia is reported to be 1–5%, with most events occurring within 10 years of treatment. However, the risk of a second solid tumor was 7.3% at 20 years and 23.5% at 30 years after treatment in a recently reported series. Approaches to decreasing these problems include decreasing or eliminating radiation therapy, omitting drugs associated with the development of leukemias, decreasing the cumulative doses of individual drugs by using multiple different drug combinations, and decreasing chemotherapy by tailoring the duration of chemotherapy to the rapidity of initial response.

References

Bhatia S, Yasui Y, Robison LL, et al. High risk of subsequent neoplasms continues with extended follow-up of childhood Hodgkin's disease: report from the late effects Study Group. J Clin Oncol. 2003;21:4386–94.

Sachellong G, Riepenhausen M, Creutzig U, et al. Low risk of secondary leukemias after chemotherapy without mechlorethamine in childhood Hodgkin's disease. J Clin Oncol. 1997;15:2247–53.

Answer to question 196: A

Educational objective

To calculate recombinant factor IX replacement dose for life-threatening bleeding in hemophilia B

Critique

Replacement factor dosing is calculated by the formula: dose factor IX (units) = units/dL (percent) desired rise in plasma factor IX × body weight (kg) × 1.0 (for factor VIII the multiplication factor is 0.5). Because of the half-life, factor VIII is administered every 10–12 h and factor IX every 20–24 h. Life-threatening bleeding episodes in hemophilia such as intracranial hemorrhage and retropharyngeal bleeding require prompt replacement of factor concentrate to a level of 100%. To calculate this dose for hemophilia A (factor VIII deficiency), 50 U/kg is given, whereas for hemophilia B (factor IX deficiency) a dose of 100 U/kg is given for plasma-derived factor IX and that dose times a factor of 1.3 for recombinant factor IX (because of a lower recovery of recombinant factor IX compared with plasma-derived factor IX). One always rounds the dose needed to the vial size, which is usually packaged in increments of 250 U; hence, 2500 U of recombinant factor IX should be given.

Reference

Montgomery RR, Gill JC, Scott JP. Hemophilia and von Willebrand disease. In: Nathan DG, Orkin SH, Ginsburg D, Look AT, eds. Nathan and Oski's Hematology of Infancy and Childhood. W.B. Saunders, 2003:1547–76.

Answer to question 197: C

Educational objective

To recognize the clinical and laboratory features of aplastic crisis in a child with a chronic hemolytic anemia

Critique

The term 'crisis' was coined to describe an acute event that disrupts the usual steady state in persons with sickle cell disease. The aplastic crisis is characterized by an episode of pure red cell aplasia resulting from the lytic action of parvovirus B19 on erythroblasts. The parvovirus attaches to the erythroblast P antigen (its receptor) and destroys the cell. Within 7–10 days these patients develop an antibody response and neutralize the virus, allowing for recovery of marrow function. Lifelong immunity ensues. Treatment includes packed red blood cell transfusion. Although this patient has mild splenomegaly (often seen in infants with sickle cell anemia), the absent reticulocyte response rules against this being splenic sequestration. A 'megaloblastic crisis' secondary to folate deficiency is very rare. This clinical scenario does not fit with vaso-occlusive crisis. Accelerated hemolysis would be extremely uncommon with a very low reticulocyte count.

Reference

Serjeant GR, Serjeant BE. Sickle Cell Disease, 3rd edn. Oxford University Press, 2001:96–104.

Answer to question 198: C

Educational objective

To recognize the potential side-effects of DDAVP in a child

Critique

Hyponatremia and possible seizures are potentially worrisome complications of DDAVP in small children and the elderly, and may occur commonly if one does not pay attention to proper fluid management. Additionally, normal children and adults may experience hyponatremia if they drink excessive free water and caffeinated beverages. Thrombosis is a rare complication and occurs mostly among middle-aged adults and the elderly. Tachyphylaxis is rare in VWD and more common in patients with hemophilia.

References

Dunn AL, Powers JR, Ribeiro MJ, Rickles, FR, Abshire TC. Adverse events during use of intranasal desmopressin acetate for mild hemophilia A and von Willebrand disease: a case report and review of forty patients. Haemophilia. 2000;6:11–4.

Smith TJ, Gill JC, Ambruso DR, Hathaway WE. Hyponatremia and seizures in young children given DDAVP. Am J Hematol. 1989;31:199–202.

Answer to question 199: E

Educational objective

To diagnose hemoglobin E and concomitant α thalassemia

Critique

The child most likely has inherited a heterozygous α mutation from one of the parents. Family studies would be confirmatory. The mild anemia, microcytosis and predominance of hemoglobin A on the hemoglobin electrophoresis exclude homozygous hemoglobin E disease and both forms of hemoglobin E β thalassemia (β^o and β^+). Although patients with hemoglobin E trait have borderline microcytosis, target cells, as well as a lower than expected percentage of hemoglobin E on electrophoresis (because of the thalassemia-like nature of the β globin gene mutation), the finding of hemoglobin E of less than 28–30% of the total hemoglobin is indicative of concomitant α thalassemia. Iron deficiency, although not listed as a choice, is unlikely in view of her normal diet.

References

Glader BE, Look KA. Hematologic disorders in children from Southeast Asia. Pediatr Clin North Am. 1996;43:665–81.

Tyagi S, Pati HP, Choudry VP, Saxena R. Clinico-haematological profile of Hb E syndrome in adults and children. Hematology. 2004;9:57–60.

Answer to question 200: C

Educational objective

To manage acute chest syndrome in a patient with hemoglobin SC disease

Critique

Patients with Hb SC and Hb S/β^+ thalassemia, in addition to patients with Hb SS, are at risk for the acute chest syndrome. Any chest symptoms should alert the clinician to this possibility. Red blood cell transfusion is beneficial for sickle cell patients with progressive lung findings and significant hypoxemia. The higher hemoglobin levels typically associated with hemoglobin SC and hemoglobin S/β^+ thalassemia, compared with Hb SS, preclude simple transfusion to substantially reduce the Hb S concentration. Exchange transfusion techniques provide red cells containing Hb A while avoiding the hyperviscosity associated with raising the Hb level above 12 g/dL. If performed manually, several units of blood need to be removed over a short period of time to provide an opportunity to transfuse an adequate amount of Hb A-containing red blood cells. Thus, manual exchange is an inefficient option. A reasonable exchange transfusion goal is to reduce the Hb S-containing cells below 30%; for Hb SC disease the fractions of both Hb S and Hb C need to be taken into consideration resulting in the target of 15% Hb S. Administration of intravenous fluids without transfusion would not be sufficient to treat acute chest syndrome with the respiratory compromise noted in this patient.

References

NIH Publication no. 02–2117. The Management of Sickle Cell Disease, 4th edn. June 2002:103–110.

Telen MJ. Principles and problems of transfusion in sickle cell disease. Semin Hematol. 2001;38:315–23.

Vichinsky EP, Neumayr LD, Earles AN, Williams R, Lennette ET, Dean D, et al. Causes and outcomes of the acute chest syndrome in sickle cell disease. National Acute Chest Syndrome Study Group. N Engl J Med. 2000;342:1855–65.

Answer to question 201: C

Educational objective

To manage hereditary spherocytosis in a patient with multiple complications

Critique

This 17-year-old has already suffered multiple complications related to hereditary spherocytosis (HS) including aplastic crisis, cholelithiasis and symptomatic anemia. Because of high levels of unconjugated bilirubin, an increased incidence of gallstones is observed in HS. In this individual with multiple episodes of right upper quadrant pain and known gallstones, cholecystectomy is indicated. The risk for common bile duct stones is higher in patients undergoing cholecystectomy without performing a concomitant splenectomy. Although splenectomy does not alter the red cell membrane abnormality of HS, reduced hemolysis will result and anemia will improve after the procedure. This patient has moderate symptomatic anemia, which is interfering with his ability to participate in high school athletics. A concomitant splenectomy is therefore indicated because of both the risk of common bile duct stones, as well as ongoing symptomatic anemia. He should receive pneumococcal, *Haemophilus influenzae* type B and meningococcal vaccines prior to the procedure. Laparoscopic surgery is preferred if possible. Medical management including increasing the dosage of folic acid would be ineffective in treating the anemia as he is already able to mount an adequate reticulocyte count. In addition, folic acid would have no impact on the risk of recurrent episodes of cholelithiasis.

Reference

Bolton-Maggs PH. The diagnosis and management of hereditary spherocytosis. Best Pract Res Clin Haematol. 2000;13:327–42.